Health Promotion in Children and Adolescents through Sport and Physical Activities—2nd Edition

Health Promotion in Children and Adolescents through Sport and Physical Activities—2nd Edition

Editor

Antonino Bianco

MDPI • Basel • Beijing • Wuhan • Barcelona • Belgrade • Manchester • Tokyo • Cluj • Tianjin

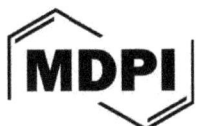

Editor
Antonino Bianco
Department of Psychology,
Educational Science and Human
Movement
University of Palermo
PALERMO
Italy

Editorial Office
MDPI
St. Alban-Anlage 66
4052 Basel, Switzerland

This is a reprint of articles from the Special Issue published online in the open access journal *Journal of Functional Morphology and Kinesiology* (ISSN 2411-5142) (available at: www.mdpi.com/journal/jfmk/special_issues/adolescents_sport_2).

For citation purposes, cite each article independently as indicated on the article page online and as indicated below:

LastName, A.A.; LastName, B.B.; LastName, C.C. Article Title. *Journal Name* **Year**, *Volume Number*, Page Range.

ISBN 978-3-0365-1197-9 (Hbk)
ISBN 978-3-0365-1196-2 (PDF)

© 2021 by the authors. Articles in this book are Open Access and distributed under the Creative Commons Attribution (CC BY) license, which allows users to download, copy and build upon published articles, as long as the author and publisher are properly credited, which ensures maximum dissemination and a wider impact of our publications.

The book as a whole is distributed by MDPI under the terms and conditions of the Creative Commons license CC BY-NC-ND.

Contents

About the Editor . . . . **vii**

Preface to "Health Promotion in Children and Adolescents through Sport and Physical Activities—2nd Edition" . . . . **ix**

Antonino Bianco
Preface to "Health Promotion in Children and Adolescents through Sport and Physical Activities—2nd Edition"
Reprinted from: *Journal of Functional Morphology and Kinesiology* 2021, 6, 23, doi:10.3390/jfmk6010023 . . . . **1**

Kwok W Ng, Fiona McHale, Karen Cotter, Donal O'Shea and Catherine Woods
Feasibility Study of the Secondary Level Active School Flag Programme: Study Protocol
Reprinted from: *Journal of Functional Morphology and Kinesiology* 2019, 4, 16, doi:10.3390/jfmk4010016 . . . . **3**

Iván Chulvi-Medrano, Manuel Pombo, Miguel Ángel Saavedra-García, Tamara Rial Rebullido and Avery D Faigenbaum
A 47-Year Comparison of Lower Body Muscular Power in Spanish Boys: A Short Report
Reprinted from: *Journal of Functional Morphology and Kinesiology* 2020, 5, 64, doi:10.3390/jfmk5030064 . . . . **23**

Josip Karuc and Marjeta Mišigoj-Duraković
Relation between Weight Status, Physical activity, Maturation, and Functional Movement in Adolescence: An Overview
Reprinted from: *Journal of Functional Morphology and Kinesiology* 2019, 4, 31, doi:10.3390/jfmk4020031 . . . . **29**

Nemanja Lakićević
The Effects of Alcohol Consumption on Recovery Following Resistance Exercise: A Systematic Review
Reprinted from: *Journal of Functional Morphology and Kinesiology* 2019, 4, 41, doi:10.3390/jfmk4030041 . . . . **37**

Avery D. Faigenbaum, Jie Kang, Nicholas A. Ratamess, Anne C. Farrell, Mina Belfert, Sean Duffy, Cara Jenson and Jill Bush
Acute Cardiometabolic Responses to Multi-Modal Integrative Neuromuscular Training in Children
Reprinted from: *Journal of Functional Morphology and Kinesiology* 2019, 4, 39, doi:10.3390/jfmk4020039 . . . . **55**

Pedro Migliano, Laura S. Kabiri, Megan Cross, Allison Butcher, Amy Frugé, Wayne Brewer and Alexis Ortiz
Validation of Cardiorespiratory Fitness Measurements in Adolescents
Reprinted from: *Journal of Functional Morphology and Kinesiology* 2019, 4, 44, doi:10.3390/jfmk4030044 . . . . **69**

Mustafa Söğüt, Ömer Barış Kaya, Kübra Altunsoy, Cain C. T. Clark, Filipe Manuel Clemente and Ali Ahmet Doğan
Anthropometric Obesity Indices, Body Fat Percentage, and Grip Strength in Young Adults with different Physical Activity Levels
Reprinted from: *Journal of Functional Morphology and Kinesiology* **2019**, 4, 51, doi:10.3390/jfmk4030051 79

Clare M. P. Roscoe, Rob S. James and Michael J. Duncan
Accelerometer-Based Physical Activity Levels Differ between Week and Weekend Days in British Preschool Children
Reprinted from: *Journal of Functional Morphology and Kinesiology* **2019**, 4, 65, doi:10.3390/jfmk4030065 87

Ludovica Gasbarro, Elvira Padua, Virginia Tancredi, Giuseppe Annino, Michela Montorsi, Grazia Maugeri and Agata Grazia D'Amico
Joint Mobility Protection during the Developmental Age among Free Climbing Practitioners: A Pilot Study
Reprinted from: *Journal of Functional Morphology and Kinesiology* **2020**, 5, 14, doi:10.3390/jfmk5010014 99

Ewan Thomas, Marianna Alesi, Garden Tabacchi, Carlos Marques da Silva, David J. Sturm, Fatma Neşe Şahin, Özkan Güler, Manuel Gómez-López, Simona Pajaujiene, Michele Basile, Ante Rada, Antonio Palma and Antonino Bianco
Cognitive and Physical Activity-Related Aspects of Children Associated to the Performance of the Crunning Movement
Reprinted from: *Journal of Functional Morphology and Kinesiology* **2021**, 6, 9, doi:10.3390/jfmk6010009 111

Terence Chua, Abdul Rashid Aziz and Michael Chia
Four Minutes of Sprint Interval Training Had No Acute Effect on Improving Alertness, Mood, and Memory of Female Primary School Children and Secondary School Adolescents: A Randomized Controlled Trial
Reprinted from: *Journal of Functional Morphology and Kinesiology* **2020**, 5, 92, doi:10.3390/jfmk5040092 123

Tamara Rial Rebullido, Cinta Gómez-Tomás, Avery D. Faigenbaum and Iván Chulvi-Medrano
The Prevalence of Urinary Incontinence among Adolescent Female Athletes: A Systematic Review
Reprinted from: *Journal of Functional Morphology and Kinesiology* **2021**, 6, 12, doi:10.3390/jfmk6010012 135

About the Editor

Antonino Bianco

Antonino Bianco (41 years old) is living in Palermo, Italy. He grew up in Resuttano (CL), a little town located in the middle of Sicily. Prof. Bianco is married to Esamuela Pieretta Mancuso and the Father of Barbara Alison Bianco. He graduated from Palermo University in Sport and Exercise Sciences; afterwards, he received a Ph.D. in Exercise Physiology (University of Palermo Medical School) and a Post-Doc in Exercise Physiology from Greenwich University (UK). He has worked for Palermo University since December 2008, and he has been an Associate Professor at the University of Palermo since November 2019. He has co-authored more than 150 peer-reviewed articles, including the GSSI Sports Nutrition Award at ECSS 2017. Of interest is that, at the age of 39, he was included within the list of the top Italian scientists in Sport and Exercise Sciences. His main research interests include: pediatric exercise and cognitive functions development; fundamentals of training methodology for muscle hypertrophy.

Preface to "Health Promotion in Children and Adolescents through Sport and Physical Activities—2nd Edition"

The second edition of the Special Issue entitled "Health Promotion in Children and Adolescents through Sport and Physical Activities"has been successfully completed, as expected. As stated in the preface to the first edition, this Special Issue (SI) was initially intended to address a challenge in this field, but this over time topic is becoming an important cornerstone for scientists who are exploring the fascinating subject of pediatric exercise. I'm grateful to all contributors for choosing MPDI and in particular my Special Issue.

Antonino Bianco
Editor

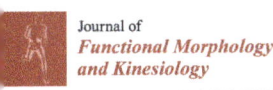

Editorial

Preface to "Health Promotion in Children and Adolescents through Sport and Physical Activities—2nd Edition"

Antonino Bianco

Sport and Exercise Sciences Research Unit, University of Palermo, Via Giovanni Pascoli, 6, 90144 Palermo, Italy; antonino.bianco@unipa.it

The second edition of the Special Issue entitled "Health Promotion in Children and Adolescents through Sport and Physical Activities" has been successfully completed, as expected. As stated in the preface to the first edition, this special issue (SI) was initially intended to address a challenge in this field, but this topic is becoming, over time, an important cornerstone for scientists who are exploring the fascinating subject of pediatric exercise. We open the second edition of this Special Issue with an interesting study protocol described by Ng et al., from the Health Research Institute, University of Limerick. The manuscript presents a useful overview of initiatives designed to encourage people to become more active and increase their awareness of the potential benefits of physical activity (PA). Chulvi-Medrano et al. present a 47-year comparison of lower body muscular power in Spanish boys. The authors conclude that a decline in lower body muscular power occurs in 10–11-year-old Spanish boys, which may be due to the increasing prevalence of sedentary lifestyles across Europe, particularly in the southern regions. Josip Karuc and Marjeta Mišigoj-Duraković investigate the relationship between functional movement (FM) patterns, PA level, and weight status in an average adolescent population. As expected, the authors reinforce the consensus that overweight and obese adolescents exhibit poorer functional movement than normal-weight adolescents. Nemanja Lakicevic, a PhD student from Palermo University, presents evidence of the effects of alcohol consumption on recovery following resistance exercise. The systematic review was publicized on social media and provides an interesting overview of the potentially negative effects of alcohol, particularly in regard to adolescents.

The acute cardiometabolic responses to multi-modal integrative neuromuscular training are reported by a pioneer in the science of modern pediatric exercise. Prof. Avery Faigenbaum is currently regarded as a major contributor in the field, often proposing new ideas and highlighting resistance training as the driving force behind the proper growth and development of coming generations. In line with Faigenbaum et al., Migliano et al. significantly contribute to this SI with their validation of cardiorespiratory fitness measurements in adolescents living in Texas (USA). Mustafa Söğüt et al. report interesting data regarding anthropometric obesity indices, body fat percentage, and grip strength in young adults. Of interest, Roscoe et al. investigate accelerometer-based physical activity levels in British preschoolers. On the other hand, joint mobility among young people participating in free climbing has been investigated by Gasbarro et al.

The ESA Program is also discussed in this Special Issue, in the contribution of Ewan Thomas et al., who consider the entire consortium involved in this innovative and sustainable European project (more than 60 people involved). The randomized controlled trial carried out by Chua et al. shows that four minutes of sprint interval training has no acute positive effects on alertness, mood, and memory in children. The study also provides useful information for physical education teachers interested in introducing new settings and scenarios to their lessons. The closing paper of the Special Issue is that by Tamara Rial and colleagues. Their investigation considers urinary incontinence (UI) among adolescent female athletes. Interestingly, the prevalence of UI among such athletes participating in impact sports was most dominant and higher in those engaged in trampolining, followed by rope skipping. In conclusion, I wish to thank the MDPI Editorial Office, and particularly Molly Lu, for supporting me in the role of SI editor. I am also grateful to the EIC Giuseppe Musumeci for the valuable guidance he provided following several rejections.

This Special Issue presents a total of 12 papers, encompassing 31 different affiliations, with authors from 12 different countries spanning three different regions of the world (Europe, North America, and Asia).

I hope to continue the success of this Special Issue with a third edition in the near future.

Conflicts of Interest: The authors declare no conflict of interest.

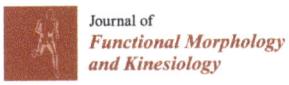

Protocol

Feasibility Study of the Secondary Level Active School Flag Programme: Study Protocol

Kwok W Ng [1,2,*], Fiona McHale [1], Karen Cotter [3], Donal O'Shea [4] and Catherine Woods [1]

[1] Department of Physical Education and Sport Sciences; Centre of Physical Activity and Health Research; Health Research Institute, University of Limerick, V94 T9PX Limerick, Ireland; fiona.mchale@ul.ie (F.M.); catherine.woods@ul.ie (C.W.)
[2] School of Educational Sciences and Psychology, University of Eastern Finland, 80101 Joensuu, Finland
[3] Active Schools Flag, Mayo Education Centre, F23 HX48 Castlebar, Ireland; karen@activeschoolflag.ie
[4] St. Vincent's University Hospital, University College Dublin, D04 T6F4 Dublin, Ireland; info@dosheaendo.ie
* Correspondence: kwok.ng@ul.ie or kwok.ng@uef.fi; Tel.: +358-50-472-4051

Received: 27 February 2019; Accepted: 19 March 2019; Published: 26 March 2019

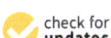

Abstract: Taking part in regular physical activity (PA) is important for young adolescents to maintain physical, social and mental health. Schools are vibrant settings for health promotion and the complexity of driving a whole-school approach to PA has not been tested in the Irish school context. The feasibility of the pilot programme of the Department of Education and Skills second level Active School Flag (SLASF) is needed. SLASF is a two year process that consists of the Active School Flag (ASF) certificate programme (year 1) and the ASF flag programme (year 2). This protocol paper is specific to the first year certificate process. Three schools around Ireland were recruited as pilot schools to carry out the year-long SLASF programme with 17 planned actions involving the entire school. Students in the transition year programme have a particular role in the promotion of PA in SLASF. Data collection consists of physical measures, accelerometers, survey data and interviews at the beginning and the end of the academic year. The primary focus on the feasibility of the programme is through process evaluation tools and fidelity checks consisting of implementation of the SLASF programme through whole-school surveys, focus group discussions of key stakeholder groups, as well as one-to-one interviews with a member of management at each school and the SLASF coordinator of the school. Secondary outcomes include PA levels and its social cognitive theories based correlates through physical health measures, surveys carried out pre- and post-intervention, as well as focus group discussions of the students. The results of this study are needed to improve the development of the SLASF through a predetermined stopping criteria and inclusion into systems thinking approaches such as the Healthy Ireland Demonstration Project.

Keywords: physical activity; adolescent; health promotion; activePal; intervention

1. Introduction

There are multiple reasons—physical, psychological, social, environmental—health for adolescents to take part in regular physical activity (PA). However, adolescence forms a highly volatile stage in life where transitional periods can influence behaviour [1] and is a critical time for PA participation where habits—good or bad—developed, later persist into adulthood [2]. Despite the evidence of health benefits from PA, a clear reduction in PA levels is apparent alongside increasing age in adolescence. Data from the Children's Sport Participation and Physical Activity (CSPPA) study highlighted a decline in meeting the PA guidelines, at least 60 min of moderate-to-vigorous (MVPA) per day, from 18% among 12y olds (first year of second level education in Ireland) to 6% among 18y olds (last year of second level education in Ireland) [3]. Similarly, a systematic review and pooled analysis indicated that PA levels decline by a mean of 7% per year over this period [4,5]. By the age of 15y, on average, across 42 countries in the Health Behaviour in School-aged Children study, only 11% of girls and 21% of boys self-reported sufficient MVPA levels [6]. Global PA decline throughout adolescence, across a range of measurement units, appears as high as 60–70% [4]. Action is needed to reduce the drop in PA levels.

Actions that target the drop in PA levels can include interventions at the individual, community and within policy [7]. Although policy interventions may provide the best return on investment [8], creating such changes requires a strong evidence base that interventions targeting the behaviours actually works. At the individual level, interventions that were designed to increase school-based PA levels have yet to demonstrate its effectiveness [8]. In particular, multi-component PA interventions have yet to demonstrate improvements in overall MVPA [9]. However, at the community level, school-based PA programmes have demonstrated some positive effect on overall PA levels [10].

1.1. Whole-School Approaches to Physical Activity Promotion

Successfully run school-based PA programmes includes quality physical education, physical activities before-, during- and after-school, at the school grounds, as well as activities based in the local community [11]. Haapala and colleagues [11] suggested that recess time activities before, during and after school are opportune moments to promote PA. Similarly, a study based on a 12 week walking intervention among girls who took part before-school and during recess times increased the time in light intensity PA by 10 min but differences in MVPA were not statistically significant when compared to the intervention group [12]. Some recent studies have investigated the role of peers in boosting PA levels. For example, peer leaders (15–16y olds) slightly older than the target group (13–15y olds) encouraged after-school activities. By the end of the 7-week after-school intervention, there was a statistically significant increase of three minutes of daily MVPA [13]. Same-aged peers were also effective in promoting six minutes of daily MVPA through diffusion messages among girls during the entire school day [14]. Statistically significant changes on PA levels were found for those identified as low active at baseline in an intervention that focused on increasing step count in both boys and girls [15]. Few school-based programmes managed to succeed in increasing boys' PA levels for school-based interventions through a peer-led model [16,17]. Programmes with in-class activities that promote PA by the class teachers are another way to increase PA levels [18]. The latter activities requires a whole-school approach towards PA promotion and in Ireland, this is known as the Active School Flag (ASF) [19].

The ASF (www.activeschoolflag.ie) is a Department of Education and Skills (DES) initiative supported by Healthy Ireland. It takes a 'whole-school approach' and requires all members of the school community to work together to strengthen the delivery of the physical education programme and to promote PA throughout the school in a fun and inclusive manner. It emphasises quality PE, co-curricular PA as well as partnerships with students, parents and the wider community. In 2018, 29% (N = 1329) of primary schools in Ireland had achieved ASF status. Some have the need for renewal, thus at the time of print, 722 primary schools currently have possession of an Active Flag. The journey towards achieving this status begins with self-evaluation in the areas of (i) physical education (ii) PA and (iii) partnerships. Following this, schools are expected to devise a strategic plan and implement changes to help improve the quality of PE, provide additional opportunities for PA and support additional involvement with the wider community. Lastly, the school has to provide a week-long focus on PA in an Active School Week.

The ASF is well-established as a primary school initiative but has yet to be developed for the secondary level education sector. A generic model has been tried among secondary level schools, although it did not achieve the same effect because the uptake of secondary level schools is below 5%. The most notable differences were the lack of whole-school engagement in the secondary level schools. Feedback from those experiences suggested that the generic ASF in secondary level was viewed as a physical education programme as opposed to a whole-school initiative. Furthermore, there are structural differences between primary and secondary level schools, thus a direct translation of the primary ASF to the secondary level setting would be specious. Some examples of differences include; in primary schools, a single teacher generally remains with the same class throughout the entire day, whereas at secondary level schools, students are taught by multiple teachers. In the secondary level schools, many schools do not have a compulsory timetabled physical education in accordance with DES recommendations (i.e., a double timetabled period for all students every week). Secondary level schools tend to be larger and cater for more students than primary schools, yet facilities for promoting PA can be limiting. Peer influences tend to be stronger at secondary level education [20] and students will often choose to socialise with their friends and be sedentary rather than take part in PA [21]. In primary schools, all teachers are encouraged to take part in continuous professional development (CPD) as part of their classroom responsibility in the areas of physical education and PA. Class teachers in secondary level schools tend to be specialists in their subject area and may not have the confidence or competence to create active breaks in the classroom [22].

In the majority of Irish secondary level schools, there is the 'Transition Year' (TY) period, whereby it is non- examinable and students may go on to try out activities beyond the normal school curriculum [23]. The aims of TY are to "increase social awareness and social competence with 'education through experience of adult and working life' as a basis for personal development and maturity" [24]. TY programmes can cover various aspects of personal development, including visits to hospitals to learn about health behaviours [25], as well as taking part in other science programmes [26]. Many TY based programmes seek to develop youth leadership skills (i.e., Gaisce the President's Award, Young Social Innovators, Gaelic Athletic Association (GAA) future leaders, etc.).

1.2. Theoretical Background to the Study

The theoretical premise of this feasibility study is underpinned by social cognitive theories [27] These theories are the most cited for health behaviour change interventions [28]. In these theories, there is a triad relationship between personal and environmental factors with behaviours being explored through individual level factors such as self-efficacy, stages of readiness for behavioural change and school related autonomy. In self-efficacy theory [29] there are four sources; mastery accomplishments, vicarious experiences, verbal persuasion and physiology are strong predictors of behaviour. Novice learners, such as students in TY, tend to have low confidence to promote PA at the beginning of the year [30]. When schools express their interest to be an SLASF school, a resource pack (see methods section) would support these students to improve the self-efficacy (opportunities for mastery accomplishments), create timetabled meetings with the purpose to focus on the SLASF (opportunities for vicarious experiences) and regular contact with others who are also carrying out the SLASF (opportunities for verbal persuasions), the sources of self-efficacy may create a better suited environment for promoting PA.

Being autonomous in making decisions is known to be directly related to intrinsic motivations towards a behaviour [31]. However, in the school context, students may feel their overall autonomy is restricted to the bounds of the school. As a result, some students may find the school environment something that they can thrive in, whereas others may feel the environment restricts individual choices. The autonomy supportive environment is as important as having autonomy among school-aged children because it can lead to greater levels of PA outside of the school context [32]. Factors that may influence the autonomy or autonomy support can include the perception of school academic performance and the way teachers and peers support academic performance [33], perceptions of ability to make decisions in the school [34] and feelings of belonging in the school [35]. Furthermore, it has been reported that individual well-being is associated with individual's sense of autonomy [36], therefore studies may need to consider the mediating factors of student well-being.

The levels of readiness for taking part in regular PA would vary vastly among the students throughout the school. According to the transtheoretical model [37] individuals are at different stages of their intention for behavioural change. Progression between the five noted stages include pre-contemplation (not ready), contemplation (getting ready), preparation (ready), action and maintenance. According to the model, the factors that influence moving between these stages consist of biopsychosocial factors, including self-efficacy, own and socially supported decisions and going through the process of change [38]. Through awareness of the stages of change among the target population, there is a greater understanding of how to create targeted interventions for the promotion of PA.

1.3. Measures of Feasibility

The SLASF programme is in its pilot phase as part of a larger systems based Healthy Ireland Demonstration Project. It is also a feasibility study, because we aim to investigate whether it is suitable in secondary level schools and if so, how to do that [39]. According to Bowen and colleagues [40], designing feasibility studies can have eight areas of focus; acceptability, demand, implementation, practicality, adaptation, integration, expansion and limited efficacy. Although the SLASF is a non-clinical study, the feasibility study is useful to provide an indicator for stopping, revisions or continuing for a scaling up a randomised control trial [41]. Moreover, the predefined rules need to be put in place prior to the analysis to prevent uncontrollable biases [42]. In Table 1, Bowen and colleagues' areas of foci for this feasibility study are broken down into the areas which this study researches and stopping criteria.

Table 1. Areas of focus for feasibility studies with measures and stopping criteria.

Focus	Measures	Stopping Criteria
Acceptability	Pragmatic survey instrument on suitability, satisfying and attractiveness for SLASF in schools for the TY and the whole-school at the end of the year.	When less than half the school students and TY consider SLASF to be suitable, satisfying or attractive to them.
	Focus group and interviews to describe the process of satisfaction of the programme, fit into the school's culture and the positive and negative effect on the school.	When interviews describe strong statements that have a negative impact on the school's culture or too much dissatisfaction to the programme.
Demand	PA audit of sections of the school.	No improvement over the academic year.
	Attendance list at the specific activities	Unsustainable numbers in attendance.
	Survey instrument based on readiness for PA behaviours.	Over half of students increased their readiness if they can.
	Focus groups based on the TY engagement in the SLASF process.	Discussions confirm low attendance rates and lack of demand for activities.
Implementation	Action Logs from the logbook.	Over half actions left incomplete
	Focus groups on implementation ease	Discussions where respondents report too many challenges preventing implementation
	Staff interviews	Data that suggests lack of resources to implement the programme and failures to execute the actions.
Practicality	Action plans for promotion of PA	If action plans could not be drawn up by the specified time frame
Adaptation	Registrations at events carried out as part of the action plan	Substantial decrease in participation over a 6 week period
Integration	Pre- and post-test results on PA opportunities and its participation	No increased opportunities since the beginning of the programme.
	Interviews with management about costs to organization and school policies	Descriptions whereby the costs are not sustainable. Indicators that there is a lack of staff
Expansion	Interviews of management	Descriptions of the uniqueness of the programme to the school and difficulties to roll out to other schools.
Limited Efficacy	Pre- and post-test results from the comprehensive surveys	Reduction in main outcome variables over the course of the year that is greater than the difference between each year cohort at the baseline measurements
	ASF logbook entries	Notes that report barriers to completing actions that are not manageable
	PA audit	Low level of usage when compared with the beginning of the year

1.4. Purpose of the Study

The primary objective for this study is to see if the SLASF certificate is an acceptable programme in secondary level Irish schools. The secondary objectives are to see how feasible it is to operationalise the components needed for testing a year-long intervention. These include collecting accelerometer and physical health measures of students in the schools, completion of survey questions for pre- and post-intervention evaluation and investigate areas for improvement from a pilot study to scale-up intervention programme.

2. Methods and Design

2.1. Setting

Eligible schools include secondary level schools in the Republic of Ireland that have not previously applied for the SLASF. Special educational needs schools or schools without a range of students from each year group are excluded. The feasibility study will be conducted in three secondary level schools, covering the demographics of a girls only school, a mixed school with designated 'Delivering Equality of Opportunity in Schools' (DEIS) status and a mixed mainstream school. A DEIS school is part of the Department of Education and Skill's action plan for educational inclusion to address disadvantaged education.

2.2. Recruitment

2.2.1. School Recruitment

The SLASF programme is a comprehensive programme and employs a whole school approach. As an intervention programme, schools were invited to take part if they are not currently in the process of obtaining the Active School Flag. The normal process of the SLASF recruitment is for schools to make an application but this was suspended to allow time to develop the new model. Schools that were interested in carrying out the feasibility study contacted the Active Schools office and requested to pilot the second level programme. There were three schools that responded and accepted because they each have a strong well-being structure in place in their schools. This is a feasibility study with secondary outcomes on efficacy hence matched control schools (one girls only, one mixed and one mixed DEIS school) were recruited to take part in the survey component of the study. No reserve list was formed for this cohort but engagement of all three schools throughout the year to follow the feasibility and evaluate the SLASF process.

2.2.2. Student Recruitment

In the participating schools, there are two levels of student engagement—basic and comprehensive. Although all students are exposed to the same SLASF programme, those engaged in the SLASF Basic are required to complete less data collection measures than those in the SLASF Comprehensive. The whole school is involved in the SLASF Basic and a random class from each year group is selected to take part in the SLASF Comprehensive. Classes are known as mixed ability tutor groups. Students obtain their consent to take part in the study. Even though there may be some students who do not obtain consent or would not like to withdraw from the comprehensive aspect of the study, there is no likely reason for them to influence the feasibility of the study.

The SLASF initiative is structured to fit into the TY framework providing real and meaningful opportunities for student voice and youth leadership. A TY class would be nominated by the school as the SLASF TY class. This TY class attends classes in relation to SLASF tasks including youth leadership, mentoring and PA promotion.

2.3. Consent

All students are given information letters for their parents. The information stated the purpose of the study as well as components of the study that would involve their child. Also, the letter invites the parents to speak to their children about the study and there are contact details to the research team to answer questions the parents may have. Because of population bias from active consent, passive consent was used for all students in the basic part of the programme. The school manages the returned forms of withdrawal. This is because it is part of the whole-school process and as a feasibility of programme, schools need to be aware of how to handle withdrawal from the programme. The online survey requests the students to give their assent (if under the age of 16) or consent (if over the age of 16).

Students assigned to the comprehensive study, receive the same information sheets as the basic programme but in addition, information about the other measures that are included as part of the feasibility and process evaluation. Parents are asked to give opt in consent due to the nature of data collection (i.e., use of accelerometers). As part of Irish law, students over the age of 16 can give their own consent to take part in the study. All students were asked to opt in to be included in video recordings of interviews.

2.4. Allocation Strategy

There was no allocation strategy used to select the schools. As a feasibility study, it was important to test the SLASF in various contexts. Three contexts were chosen; a DEIS school, a girls only school and a mixed school. All schools are considered to be large in size and this would test out the possible whole-school approach.

2.5. Active School Flag Intervention

The SLASF feasibility model is co-designed by a SLASF steering group and staff, researchers of the University of Limerick and feedback from the three lead schools. The SLASF process is designed to be peer-led by a TY SLASF class, who will have the support of an SLASF coordinator, SLASF committee members, school staff and school management. The initiative challenges peers to find ways to encourage more students in their school to engage in school-based PA opportunities (year 1—SLASF certificate) and community-based PA opportunities (year 2—SLASF flag). During year 1 (Active School Flag certificate) the focus is on increasing participation in school-based PA opportunities. Year 2 (Active School Flag) is focused on community-based activities.

Previously the SLASF was viewed as a physical education initiative. In order to generate greater whole-school engagement, the SLASF tasks are formatted to draw support for the SLASF TY team from school management and teachers across a variety of different subjects. The new format of the SLASF process complements two current key educational initiatives: The Well-Being Framework by the Irish National Council for Curriculum and Assessment, the School Self-Evaluation process by the Department of Education and Skills and a new initiative presently at draft stage: The Parent and Student Charter also by the Department of Education and Skills. Students working towards Gaisce the President's Award can use their SLASF work to fulfil their Community or Personal Skill challenge requirement. Another benefit of SLASF is that it will link schools with the current national Healthy Ireland PA programmes and national youth charity events including:

- Get Ireland Walking—www.getirelandwalking.ie
- Parkrun—www.parkrun.ie
- Get Ireland Swimming—www.swimireland.ie/get-swimming
- Swim for a Mile Challenge—www.swimireland.ie/get-swimming/swim-for-a-mile
- Darkness into Light—www.darknessintolight.ie
- Cycle Against Suicide—www.cycleagainstsuicide.com

The SLASF programme is a whole-school approach to increase PA opportunities and generate opportunities for student voice and youth leadership. Currently, there are two levels. The first level is a certificate. This is open to all secondary level schools. It can serve as a good link from primary schools to continue on the ethos of active schools and allow a school to consider whether to take the next step or not. Moreover, SLASF is a DES (Department of Education and Skills) initiative and it can only be awarded to schools that adhere to physical education timetable recommendations that is, a double timetabled period of physical education for all year groups. This provision is not in place in a large number of secondary level schools, thus heretofore excluding them from the SLASF process. The introduction of the certificate level, without eligibility criteria, opens the SLASF process to all interested post primary schools. If the SLASF certificate proves beneficial it may encourage them to revisit their timetable policy.

Achievement of the flag is a whole school process, meaning that management, staff and students all play a role in the programme. There is a requirement for website updates and an online presence. In order to achieve the SLASF Certificate a number of tasks must be completed during year 1. These include: (1) a staff slideshow, (2) an SLASF team slideshow, (3) class time slideshow (4) SLASF training day, (5) an SLASF awareness week (towards the beginning of the year), (6) website showcase, (7) SLASF whole school questionnaire, (8) SLASF launch event, (9) SLASF action plan, (10) 'Did You Know?' campaign, (11) PA module as part of Social, personal and health education (SPHE) subject for junior cycle students, (12) Active School WALKWAY, (13) Community Mapping of extra curriculum activities, (14) Community Event, (15) Active School Week, (16) SLASF accreditation visit and (17) school PA space audits (Figure 1).

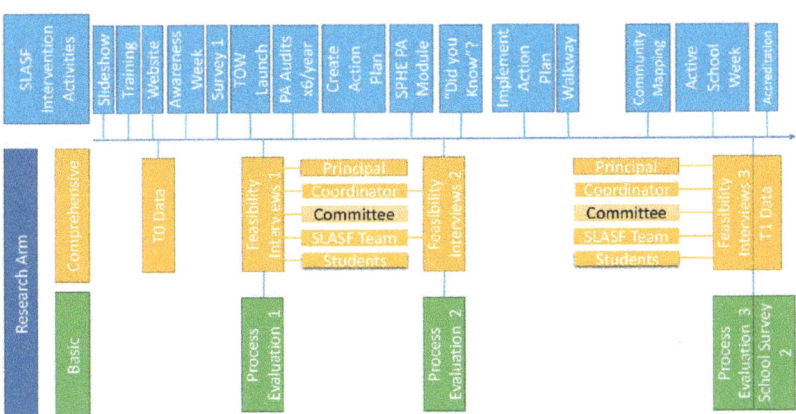

Figure 1. Second Level Active School Flag (SLASF) Intervention and Research Components Timeline.

All 17 activities are scheduled throughout the school year including a combination of staff and students as the main actors in this process. The SLASF TY class should take leadership guided and supported by the SLASF coordinator and committee on the programme. A key part of the process is that the SLASF coordinator has timetable provision allocated to two class periods per week to carry out work with the TY class. The committee includes staff representatives from the school, including one from management, an SLASF coordinator, two other staff who work on the well-being curriculum to include SPHE, Civic, Social, Political Education (CSPE) and Physical Education teachers, as well as four youth leaders. Structure of different actors in the process can be viewed in Figure 2.

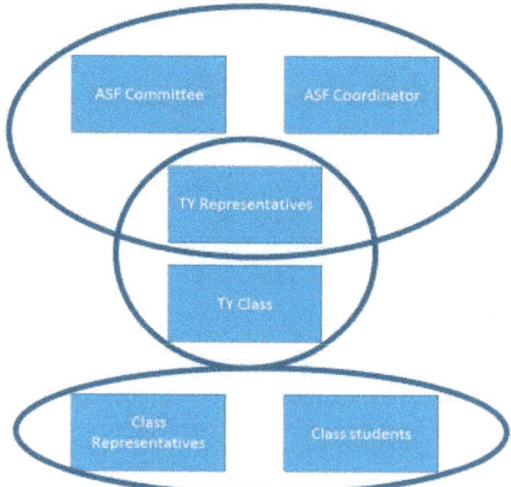

Figure 2. Actors of the Second Level Active school Flag.

Schools wishing to work towards the second level of the SLASF process, the Active School Flag, must have completed the certificate level and be able to confirm that they timetable physical education in accordance with DES recommendations.

At the student level, there are three levels of involvement. There is the SLASF team, which is comprised of the SLASF TY programme group. There are four SLASF youth leaders who represent the team at the school committee level. To be a youth leader, the SLASF team member needs to apply for the position through an application process that is evaluated by the staff members of the SLASF committee. The youth leaders end up representing the student voice at the SLASF committee and have the responsibility of presenting the SLASF action plan and the SLASF end of year review to the school Principal. The third student level is the SLASF class representatives. There are two in every class in the school and students can also apply for this position through an application form. The selection will be made by the class tutor in consultation with the SLASF coordinator.

2.5.1. TY Leader Role

The TY leader role is responsible for planning, promoting and implementing the SLASF initiatives and events throughout the school year. Based on self-efficacy theory [29], TY leaders are a closer connection to the students in the schools than teachers, thus strengthen vicarious experiences. Moreover, social support and leadership from the TYs can reinforce the basic premise of proactive behaviour change [43]. The SLASF team can be identified by being given pins to wear on their uniform. Moreover, part of the time spent on SLASF activities can be used as part of a time bank for other volunteering programmes, such as, Gaisce the President's Award. The selected SLASF youth leaders will receive their own distinct pins to wear on the uniform.

2.5.2. Activities for Certification

For schools to be successful in achieving the activities needed for certification, there is a yearly planner with guideline dates for task completion that the schools will use to keep on track. This also includes the accreditation visit. For example, the SLASF slideshows for the staff, team and youth leaders need to have been completed before the 2nd week of the school year. A designated training day takes place a week later. The purpose of this training day is to introduce the pilot schools to each other and the research team. The research team describes the whole year process evaluation and measurements taken throughout the year. There are co-design opportunities between the TY leaders and researchers to formulate the surveys used to collect data. The training day is not expected to run every year once feasibility is over. At this training day, two members of staff, the SLASF coordinator and another on the SLASF team take four student leaders to a training venue to learn about how to run the activities throughout the year. The website should also go live at the outset of the process. The website should encompass an easy to find link to the SLASF section of the site and there are the four core parts of the SLASF process; Physical Education; PA; Partnerships; and Active School Week.

- Another activity that the school needs to complete is the SLASF Awareness Week. This should be completed two weeks after the training day.
- School census questionnaire is deployed a week after the awareness week and this precedes the official launch of the SLASF process.
- During the launch, there would be a school wide tug of war (TOW) competition that is planned, promoted and organised by the SLASF committee.
- For the launch day the overall winning TOW team will compete against a staff team at a whole school event to launch the SLASF initiative.

A school census questionnaire was developed to help the SLASF team to identify their action plan. Core questions about PA opportunities, physical education, involvement in extra-curriculum activities and barriers to PA were included in an online survey. For a week after the awareness week, the survey is available for completion. All responses are anonymous and completed confidentially. Class teachers supervise and help answer any technical questions related to the completion of the survey. The data is stored on a secure server that is only accessible to the researchers. However, the overall results for each variable would be computed and provided for the school to carry out their own descriptive analyses with the TY group. The TY class can then produce meaningful findings from the survey to show the school through the notice board and used for one of the planned actions.

For the TOW event a free rope and a 2 1/2 h workshop will be provided for each school. This will enable TYs to coach and officiate TOW competitions and SLASF committee members that complete the course will receive a TOW Community Coach certificate upon completion. Each class in the school will be involved in this event with each having 3 TOW teams that compete against each other during tutor time or physical education class to decide what team will represent the class. Each class TOW team competes against the other classes in their year group during lunchtime to find the best TOW team for their year. Local role models can be invited to help launch the event by taking part in one of the TOW teams. This event should take place before the mid-autumn break.

After the mid-autumn break, the schools would have access to their school's results from the school questionnaire. The SLASF teams are given a month to review the results and start to design an SLASF action plan. At least three action points need to be agreed upon by the SLASF team. The proposed SLASF actions should be presented to the Principal for agreement. The agreed actions are then implemented in the second half of the school year. Towards the end of the year, the three agreed actions will be reviewed by the SLASF team members and presented to the school Principal during the last two weeks of the school year.

In addition, all students in the selected year group in the school will take part in a four weeks PA module delivered by the Social and Personal Health Education (SPHE) teachers. There would have to be a 'Did You Know?' campaign around the school that helps raise awareness about the benefits of PA for teenagers, in particular the positive impact that PA has upon focus, concentration and academic achievement. Another practical task for the SLASF team is to signpost an Active School WALKWAY. The walkway is a route that can be used by the students in the school during recess time or under teacher supervision for active learning activities, before/after tests or during free classes. SLASF, in partnership with Get Ireland Walking, designed Active School WALKWAY packs consisting of colourful outdoor all-weather sign post plaques which include orienteering symbols. One of the tasks that the SLASF TY class have to undertake is to map, measure and erect the walkway signposts to create a school walking route. A school WALKWAY Day where all classes get the opportunity to complete the walkway route with their teachers on a nominated school day needs to be agreed by school management. Then it is organised and promoted by the SLASF TY team. The organised walkway can be used as part of orienteering activities during timetabled physical education, as well as other school-based initiatives.

As the year ends, the school prepares for the accreditation visit for the certificate. A follow up visit takes place during the acquisition of the flag year. Prior to this, the school needs to organise a community mapping exercise and community events which should help with the design of the Active School Week (ASW) programme. The main aims of the ASW are to promote PA in a fun and inclusive way, as well as raising awareness about the availability and variety of PA opportunities for teenagers and their families in their local community. Throughout this week the school provides many and varied opportunities for staff and students to become more physically active throughout the school day.

2.5.3. Expected Outcomes Tables and Measures

According to their training resources, the programme aims to impact on a number of areas. However, to measure them all, multiple sources are required. A collection of survey instruments can be used to measure some of the outcomes, whereas some interviews can be used to evaluate other outcomes. In addition, the programme is year-long and a whole-school approach, hence site visits and checking on progress through logbook entries would be used to determine the processes carried out during the study. In Table 2, there is a list of the areas that SLASF aims to promote and some measures that can be used to test these outcomes.

Table 2. Aligning outcomes with measures.

SLASF Target Areas	Measures of Efficacy	Details
Physically educated	Self-efficacy in PA	Student survey
Physically active school community	Comprehensive Survey and focus groups	Survey item and discussions
Broad physical education	Whole-school survey and focus groups	List of physical education activities and discussions
Balanced physical education	Teacher scheme of work	Teacher records
More inclusiveness	Teacher scheme of work	Teacher records
Partnership with others to promote pa culture	TY logbook	Taster session from ASW
Active school week	TY logbook	Record of entries
Increased concentration	Harter scale	Student survey
Improved learning	Teachers perceptions	Student and teacher survey
Maintenance of discipline	Teacher records	Discipline records
Improved test results	Winter and summer test	Academic records
School enjoyment	Questionnaire	Student survey
Increase Daily PA	Accelerometers	Comprehensive Data
Reduced sitting time	Accelerometers	Comprehensive Data
Reduction in overweight and obesity	Self-report and anthropometric measures of height and weight	Comprehensive data

2.5.4. Questionnaires

There are two types of online surveys carried out throughout the year. The basic survey is completed by the entire school. This survey is anonymous and the focus is on PA participation and barriers to school related physical activities. This survey is a compulsory part of the SLASF process. Administration of the survey is decided by the school, with the intention to cover the entire school. Ideally, a census sweep of the school takes place at the same time. However, there may be some technical issues that may prevent this from happening. For example, schools may have a limited number of computers accessing the internet at any one time (bandwidth limits), may have a limited number of units to complete the survey (lack of tablets or computers) or could not get all the school to take part at the same time (timetabling issues). The results of the survey will be given back to the school for the purpose to plan specific school-based interventions. Therefore, it is important that the mode of data collection, analysis and reporting can be completed quickly and easily. Failing all technical capabilities to collect from an online platform, extra resources would be dedicated to ensure double coding from pen and paper surveys.

The second type of survey is a comprehensive survey, used for evaluating the feasibility of the study. The participants in this study input their user-ID so that the data can be linked from the beginning and end of the year long programme. Completion of the online survey takes place as one of the testing stations during the data collection visits. All the students have tablets or allocated to a school computer to complete the online survey. Details of the instruments are reported in Table 3.

Table 3. Battery of questionnaires.

Battery	Items	Response Scales	Psychometric Information
PA Screening measure	2 items on number of days in a week of at least 60 min of MVPA per day	0–7 days	Validity & Reliability [5,44]
PA opportunities	Modified items about local opportunities for PA to the context of schools instead of 'residential area'	5 point scale, 1 = disagree a lot, 5 = agree a lot	Original items used from an interview guide.
The exercise self-efficacy scale for adolescents	10 items on confidence to participate in a variety of conditions	11 point sliding scale, 0 = not at all confident, 10 = very confident	Nigg & Courneya, 1999 [45]
PA peer support scale	4 items on the frequency of peers influence for PA	0 = never, 5 = every day	Prochaska et al., 2002 [46]
PA, plans, expectancy and intention	Modified 3 items on the planning, expectancy and intention to do PA in the coming week	1 = unlikely, 8 = likely	Hagger et al., 2001 [47]
Readiness for behaviour change	Single item to determine which stage of the transtheoretical model in terms of PA	Select one item of each stage of the transtheoretical model	Lee et al., 2001 [48]
Perceived school performance	Single item about perceptions of teacher's evaluation of students' grade	Very good, good, average, below average	Felder-Puig et al., 2012 [49]
Perceived school performance	Two items about the students perception of their school grades	5 point scale, 1 = strongly disagree, 5 = strongly agree	Felder-Puig et al., 2012 [49]
Harter's Self-perception scale for adolescents	5 items from the scholastic competence subscale.	Polarised responding	Harter et al., 1982 [50]
Belonging in school	2 items on belonging to a school	1 = Strongly agree, 5 = strongly disagree	OECD
School satisfaction	How do you feel about school a present	1 = I like it a lot, 5 = I don't like it at all	HBSC since 2001
School effort	How pressured do you feel by the schoolwork you have to do	Not at all, A little, Some, A lot	HBSC since 2001
Participation of organised activities	3 items about the student-led activities at school.	1 = Strongly agree, 5 = strongly disagree	HBSC in 2013/14
Kidscreen-27	Items on the physical and psychological well-being and the autonomy and parent relations	Not at all, Slightly, Moderately, Extremely	Ravens-Sieberer, et al., 2006 [51]

2.6. Process Evaluation

2.6.1. Logbook Activities

Each school is given a logbook to record their activities. This is used as part of the accreditation process and is used by the researchers to evaluate the processes that the school used. The logbook is mainly used by the SLASF team and the SLASF committees. Every week, the TY students have the opportunity to complete a small section in the diary to record what took place. The diary is linked to the school year and the expected timescale for carrying out specific activities. There is also a chart for the SLASF team to complete by recording the agreed actions to be carried out by the SLASF team. The team need to record the date of the agreed action, a short title for the action, the person(s) responsible, date of the action completed and a check box.

The TY team carries out a brief version of the System of Observing Play and Leisure Activity in Youth (SOPLAY) [52]. SOPLAY is a direct observation tool that is used by the TYs to assess PA levels within specific PA areas in the school. Due to resources, the full SOPLAY protocol had to be reduced down to three specific areas around the school. Furthermore, the TYs use tablets to video record the specific area and retrospectively carry out the observations. It is designed in this way because the technology is more readily available in schools than the time when SOPLAY was created by McKenzie and colleagues [52]. Through, observing the video recordings, the results can be verified so the validity of the results are stronger. Trained researchers with the SOPLAY counting system can verify the results from the TYs by matching the observation results. The videos can also be used as part of a TY class, where the students can get an understanding of ways to record the different intensities of PA. The SOPLAY exercise is carried out over six times throughout the school year. The assignment of the dates are researcher assigned days. The TYs are informed of the audit in the morning of the day the recording takes place. To reduce potential bias in the results, the TYs are reminded not to tell others that they are carrying out the observation. Observations take place twice during lunchtimes, one 10 min into the beginning and the second when there is 10 min left.

Another activity recorded in the logbook is the SLASF committee meetings. The logbook provides space for six meetings throughout the year. The meeting minutes include the people in attendance, the areas of discussion and the actions that were agreed. There is also space in the logbook has space for a list of agreed action created by the TY class during their timetabled class time. To encourage compliance, there is room for information such as the agreed action, the person responsible and the date for completion. In addition, there is room in the logbook for the TY team and coordinator to note activities that take place in a specific week. For each week, tasks that are suggested, such as the slide show, presentation of the action plan and so forth are available for the TY and coordinator to help remind to be on track.

2.6.2. Whole-School Surveys

There are three surveys to be carried out by all students in the school. The whole-school survey is part of the feasibility study and is carried out through an online survey platform. It is a mandatory action to be carried out by the school and is carried out during the first two months of the academic year. The school uses this information for creating and implementing three school specific action plans. Within this survey there are details of participation levels and barriers to taking part in physical education and extra curriculum activities. Both staff and students complete a second survey halfway through the process with items also related to process evaluation. Items will test implementation, fidelity and satisfaction of the tasks completed to date. The final whole-school survey has items related to process evaluation and is completed towards the end of the academic year but before the accreditation visit. The survey will also be held on an online survey platform. Due to the difficulties in getting whole-school engagement towards the end of the school year, the survey has pragmatic evaluation items whereby it can be completed on a mobile device such as a tablet or smart phone.

2.7. Sample Size

There are three schools that are part of the feasibility study. Unlike a sample size calculation, a justification is made for feasibility studies [53]. In Table 4, information about the size of the school, the type and the number of participants expected to complete the comprehensive arm of the study is presented.

According to the Department of Education and Skills school lists, School B is one of the largest secondary level in Ireland, with 1313 enrolled students. It is also a DEIS school. Approximately 10% of secondary level students attend a DEIS designated school. Moreover, there are known socioeconomic barriers towards PA [6], therefore it is necessary to carry out this feasibility in a DEIS school environment. School A is an all-girls school. Almost one in five schools in the country are all-girls' schools. There are many reports of girls having lower levels of PA than boys and therefore it is essential to include an all-girl's school. School C has a slightly fewer number of students than the national average of 999 students per school. Moreover, the ratio between girls and boys is slightly higher for girls (1:1.05), whereas the national average in mixed schools tends to have fewer girls than boys (1:0.87).

Table 4. Sample size descriptions.

School	Students	Girls	Boys	Teachers	DEIS	Comprehensive (N)
Intervention						
A	971	971	-	70	N	100
B	863	440	423	70	N	150
C	1313	664	649	120	Y	150
Control						
D	582	582	-	41	N	123
E	629	322	307	45	N	121
F	378	206	172	35	Y	88

2.8. Data Analyses

2.8.1. Quantitative Data

The data from the surveys are analysed through relevant statistical methods for the follow up data in this feasibility study. Compatible data between comprehensive and basic surveys can be used to determine the test-retest reliability of the items given that a smaller subsample of the entire school. As reliability is an important psychometric property for question items, this is carried out during the first phase of data collection.

Students take part in the comprehensive study have their measures taken two times during the academic year. The first time takes place in autumn 2018 and the second takes place six months later during the spring 2019. Accelerometer data are transferred through the ActivPal software based on 15sec epoch. The standardised cut-offs for different types of motion; sleep, standing, light, moderate and vigorous PA are then compared at an individual level from pre- and post-test time points. Similarly, the height, weight and grip strength data is compared between the time points and used to control the differences in accelerometer data. Comprehensive survey data is also analysed with differences in PA and school related factors.

Exploratory approaches include cross-sectional multivariate analyses of PA and school-related factors as independent variables and device-based PA and perceptions of PA opportunities as the dependent variables. Mixed models and multi-level regression analyses can be used on the data that has sufficient follow up data from the first time point. The multi-level approach takes into account between- and within- individual processes that explain variances in the outcome measures. Through this approach, it is possible to test the extent of PA (psychosocial variables) and school-related factors in relation to changes in PA levels and opportunities, at the same time to examine the individual versus the school factors that contribute to the outcome variables.

The follow-up data adds another level of analysis that can test the changes through the intervention. It makes it possible to examine, for example, the changes in PA levels across the schools from the beginning and the end of the study, while also taking into account changes in the psychosocial variables included in this study. The interactions between the contexts can confirm behavioural change theories by examining the mediating and moderation mechanisms in PA levels. The majority of the statistical analysis would be carried out using IBM SPSS.

2.8.2. Qualitative Data

The majority of the qualitative data comprises of focus group data. The way data is captured is a summary of individuals who collectively agree and discuss on the content [54]. Therefore, the first phase of analysis is to provide quantitative analysis of the subjects and the group types [55]. Focus groups can be useful to find a consensus on a phenomenon, as well as to engage with participants to discuss and share ideas that would otherwise be difficult to gather from one to one interviews [56]. In particular, the structural approach to children's group research can be used and transferred across to adolescents so that the students' voice to be heard [57]. Because the way a person in the focus group may consider a way to respond to the moderators' questions could differ from what other individuals may be thinking at the time, it is important to consider the way individuals respond, with whom and in what ways [55]. Transcriptions are matched with assistant moderator notes of verbal and non-verbal behaviours.

The data from one-to-one interviews is more straightforward. A semi-structure interview guide is used to direct the respondent to focus on the research questions and is used for further probing into these questions if the respondent needs to explain something further. Interviewees data are also merged with intonation coding to help reinforce the importance of non-verbal behaviour. The double coding from the transcription across the different qualitative approaches creates a rich source of data.

The combination of data is inserted into NVivo software for qualitative analysis. The metadata and types of data are used to create a rich data set. The data undergoes a thematic analysis as suggested by Lederman [58] by (1) identifying the big ideas, (2) creating units of data, (3) categorizing the units, (4) negotiating categories and (5) identifying themes and use of theory. The theories surrounding social-cognitive theories, including self-efficacy theory [29], self-determination theory [31] and competence motivation theory [50] are lens used in the final steps of the content analyses.

The data are collected through follow up measures throughout the year. The researchers incorporate verification checking at the beginning of each session to place a point where the respondents can focus on. In particular, we are interested in the processes of the intervention, as well as the potential transformation in beliefs, thoughts and actions over the course of the year. These steps are useful for designing the results in a way that allows for multi-method approach to the overall research questions.

2.8.3. Mixed Methods Analyses

Both quantitative and qualitative data can complement each other. We hope that the data that derives from both methods of inquiry can be partly explained through the literature to date and other types of data that is collected. To return to the points of evaluation of the feasibility study, there are various numbers of expected outcomes that the school is expected to achieve and they are measured directed through particular sources (Table 2). For example, the expected outcome of a broad physical education curriculum is measured through the whole school survey on participation of various physical education activities. The data taken from the beginning of the year gives insight to the types of activities that the students reported to have attended in the past 12 months. Through data collection across all year groups, the survey data can be used to determine how broad the physical education programme actually is. The post-test survey would give an indication of the extent of the physical education programme. However, reliance solely on this measure may be limited to the actual item that is included in the survey [59]. Therefore, combining the data from focus groups by the students and staff at the school can give more details about what was popular, who experienced the changes and the mechanisms in place to make the broader physical education opportunities. Therefore, the focus on the results are on the processes of creating the change, thus allowing further insight into the behavioural change techniques used to facilitate such changes.

The SLASF log data contains both quantitative and qualitative data and can be analysed for the percent of completion towards the SLASF. Actions in relation to SLASF throughout the year form descriptive feasibility analyses. Differences in the PA audit across the year are analysed through descriptive statistics over time. In combination with the logbook of actions and the results of the PA audit more details about the feasibility of schools' actions from the TY class can be determined in relation to desired outcomes.

2.9. Availability of Data and Materials

After completion of the study, data will be stored at the University of Limerick's Data archive without potential identifiers and request for data can be made through the study's principal investigator (Last author). All supplementary materials for the SLASF programme including the resource pack, template logbook and accompanying resources will be available at https://osf.io/frx6t/.

2.10. Ethics Approval and Consent to Participate

The study follows the principles of the Declaration of Helsinki. The study protocol has been approved by the research ethics committee of the Faculty of Education and Health Sciences, University of Limerick (ref no. 2018/10/18_EHS). Written informed consent will be sought from participating teachers, students and students' guardians. All participants have permission to withdraw from the study at any time and data deleted if collected. In cases of important protocol changes, requests from the ethical committee will be sought for. Trial Registration: https://osf.io/keubz/register/5771ca429ad5a1020de2872e; Registered 24th September 2018; Clinical Trial Registration: NCT03847831.

3. Discussion

In this year-long feasibility study of the SLASF, a mixed-method approach is used to give recommendation to stop, revise or conduct a randomised control trial. The whole-school approach requires multiple stakeholders, primarily the students in secondary level schools, the TY students, the SLASF staff and its committee, as well as the management. The theories used in this paper are based on social cognitive theories and stages of change model [29,31,50].

Whole-school based interventions in the promotion of PA have been increasing [11,19] although the inception of the SLASF in the secondary level schools is more complicated than primary level schools. The diversity of foci at secondary level schools brings challenges towards a uniform and national programme. This is evident to date, whereby 29% of primary schools are ASF schools, whereas less than 5% of secondary level schools have this status. Therefore, a feasibility study is needed to test the readiness prior to national roll-out.

The results from this study would be used to help inform the development of the SLASF and report the experiences of the schools in the feasibility study. Secondary outcomes from the measures carried out in the study may lead to improved understanding of the mechanisms of the promotion of PA. Moreover, the direct mapping of the stated goals of the SLASF with measures would provide evidence. Future iterations of the SLASF may include opt in by the students to take part in the SLASF TY programme, thus providing a mixture of students who are active and inactive.

The challenges to this programme include the fidelity of the year-long programme. Schools are dynamic systems all with different characteristics based on the people who attend it. Challenging aspects could include issues arising from the coordination of the staff and pupils to carry out the tasks. There may be other activities that take place in the school, which reduce the efforts needed to run the programme or conversely, highly engagement that roles are dispersed more than previously planned. Monitoring of fidelity and carrying out process evaluations would help inform the way the programme is run.

This feasibility study is novel in design in that it a whole-school approach to the promotion of physical activity among adolescents who are empowered to organize activities over the course of the year. School management also receive an incentive by striving towards the goal and recognition of an Active School Flag. Successful piloting of the SLASF can lead to upscaling to all secondary level schools around the Republic of Ireland due to the programme endorsement by the Department of Education and Skills. Testing of the programme can be part of large scale RCT that would fit under the Healthy Ireland Demonstration Project.

Author Contributions: K.W.N. drafted the manuscript. All authors were responsible for writing part of the manuscript and critically revising the complete manuscript. F.M. contributed to the background and concept of the study. K.C. contributed to the design of the programme. D.O. contributed to the study design. C.W. is the principal investigator and contributed to the concept and design of the study. All authors approved the final manuscript.

Funding: The feasibility study is funded by Mayo Education Centre, Healthy Ireland and St. Vincent's Foundation.

Acknowledgments: K.W.N., F.M., D.O. and C.W. are researchers who have remained independent in the design of the SLASF programme. K.C. is a member of the ASF steering committee and designed the SLASF programme. K.C.'s involvement was to ensure all the aspects of this protocol are correct. K.C. has no involvement with carrying out the research, either in data collection or analyses.

Conflicts of Interest: K.C. is employed by the Mayo Education Centre although K.C. is not involved in carrying out the research. All other authors declare that they have no competing interests.

References

1. Patton, G.C.; Sawyer, S.M.; Santelli, J.S.; Ross, D.A.; Afifi, R.; Allen, N.B.; Arora, M.; Azzopardi, P.; Baldwin, W.; Bonell, C.; et al. Our future: A Lancet commission on adolescent health and wellbeing. *Lancet* **2016**, *387*, 2423–2478. [CrossRef]
2. Telama, R. Tracking of physical activity from childhood to adulthood: A review. *Obes. Facts* **2009**, *2*, 187–195. [CrossRef] [PubMed]
3. Woods, C.B.; Tannerhill, D.; Quinlan, A.; Moyna, N.; Walsh, J. *The Children's Sport Participation and Physical Activity Study (CSPPA)*; Irish Sports Council: Dublin, Ireland, 2010.
4. Dumith, S.C.; Gigante, D.P.; Domingues, M.R.; Kohl, H.W. Physical activity change during adolescence: A systematic review and a pooled analysis. *Int. J. Epidemiol.* **2011**, *40*, 685–698. [CrossRef] [PubMed]
5. Hardie Murphy, M.; Rowe, D.A.; Woods, C.B. Impact of physical activity domain on subsequent activity in youth: A 5-year longitudinal study. *J. Sports Sci.* **2017**, *35*, 262–268. [CrossRef]
6. Inchley, J.; Currie, D.; Young, T.; Samdal, O.; Torsheim, T.; Augustson, L.; Mathison, F.; Aleman-Diaz, A.; Molcho, M.; Weber, M.; Barnekow, V. *Growing Up Unequal: Gender and Socioeconomic Differences in Young People's Health and Well-Being. Health Behaviour in School-Aged Children (HBSC) Study: International Report from the 2013/2014 Survey*; Report No.: Health Policy for Children and Adolescents, No.7; WHO Regional Office for Europe: Copenhagen, Denmark, 2016.
7. Schilling, J.M.; GilesCorti, B.; Sallis, J.F. Connecting active living research and public policy: Transdisciplinary research and policy interventions to increase physical activity. *J. Public Health Policy* **2009**, *30* (Suppl. 1), S1–S15. [CrossRef] [PubMed]
8. Masters, R.; Anwar, E.; Collins, B.; Cookson, R.; Capewell, S. Return on investment of public health interventions: A systematic review. *J. Epidemiol. Community Health* **2017**, *71*, 827–834. [CrossRef]
9. Love, R.; Adams, J.; van Sluijs, E.M.F. Are school-based physical activity interventions effective and equitable? A meta-analysis of cluster randomized controlled trials with accelerometer-assessed activity. *Obes. Rev.* **2019**. [CrossRef]
10. Pate, R.R.; Dowda, M. Raising an Active and Healthy Generation: A Comprehensive Public Health Initiative. *Exerc. Sport Sci. Rev.* **2019**, *47*, 3–14. [CrossRef]
11. Haapala, H.L.; Hirvensalo, M.H.; Laine, K.; Laakso, L.; Hakonen, H.; Kankaanpää, A.; Lintunen, T.; Tammelin, T.H. Recess physical activity and school-related social factors in Finnish primary and lower secondary schools: Cross-sectional associations. *BMC Public Health* **2014**, *14*, 1114. [CrossRef]
12. Carlin, A.; Murphy, M.H.; Nevill, A.; Gallagher, A.M. Effects of a peer-led Walking in ScHools intervention (the WISH study) on physical activity levels of adolescent girls: A cluster randomised pilot study. *Trials* **2018**, *19*, 31. [CrossRef]

13. Owen, M.B.; Kerner, C.; Taylor, S.L.; Noonan, R.J.; Newson, L.; Kosteli, M.C.; Curry, W.B.; Fairclough, S.J. The Feasibility of a Novel School Peer-Led Mentoring Model to Improve the Physical Activity Levels and Sedentary Time of Adolescent Girls: The Girls Peer Activity (G-PACT) Project. *Children* **2018**, *5*, 67. [CrossRef]
14. Sebire, S.J.; Jago, R.; Banfield, K.; Edwards, M.J.; Campbell, R.; Kipping, R.; Blair, P.S.; Kadir, B.; Garfield, K.; Matthews, J.; et al. Results of a feasibility cluster randomised controlled trial of a peer-led school-based intervention to increase the physical activity of adolescent girls (PLAN-A). *Int. J. Behav. Nutr. Phys. Act.* **2018**, *15*, 50. [CrossRef] [PubMed]
15. Lubans, D.; Morgan, P. Impact of an extra-curricular school sport programme on determinants of objectively measured physical activity among adolescents. *Health Educ. J.* **2008**, *67*, 305–320. [CrossRef]
16. Lubans, D.R.; Morgan, P.J.; Aguiar, E.J.; Callister, R. Randomized controlled trial of the Physical Activity Leaders (PALs) program for adolescent boys from disadvantaged secondary schools. *Prev. Med.* **2011**, *52*, 239–246. [CrossRef]
17. Smith, J.J.; Morgan, P.J.; Plotnikoff, R.C.; Stodden, D.F.; Lubans, D.R. Mediating effects of resistance training skill competency on health-related fitness and physical activity: The ATLAS cluster randomised controlled trial. *J. Sports Sci.* **2016**, *34*, 772–779. [CrossRef]
18. Dobbins, M.; Husson, H.; DeCorby, K.; LaRocca, R.L. School-based physical activity programs for promoting physical activity and fitness in children and adolescents aged 6 to 18. *Cochrane Database Syst. Rev.* **2013**, 2. [CrossRef]
19. McMullen, J.; Ní Chróinín, D.; Tammelin, T.; Pogorzelska, M.; van der Mars, H. International Approaches to Whole-of-School Physical Activity Promotion. *Quest* **2015**, *67*, 384–399. [CrossRef]
20. Davison, K.K.; Jago, R. Change in parent and peer support across ages 9 to 15 yr and adolescent girls' physical activity. *Med. Sci. Sports Exerc.* **2009**, *41*, 1816–1825. [CrossRef]
21. Fitzgerald, A.; Fitzgerald, N.; Aherne, C. Do peers matter? A review of peer and/or friends' influence on physical activity among American adolescents. *J. Adolesc.* **2012**, *35*, 941–958. [CrossRef]
22. Jenkinson, K.A.; Benson, A.C. Barriers to Providing Physical Education and Physical Activity in Victorian State Secondary Schools. *Aust. J. Teach. Educ.* **2010**, *35*, 1–17. [CrossRef]
23. Clerkin, A. Personal development in secondary education: The Irish transition year. *Educ. Policy Anal. Arch.* **2012**, *20*. [CrossRef]
24. Jeffers, G. The Transition Year programme in Ireland. Embracing and resisting a curriculum innovation. *Curric. J.* **2011**, *22*, 61–76. [CrossRef]
25. Kelleher, C.; Kelly, D.; Finnegan, O.; Kerley, M.; Doherty, K.; Gilroy, I.; Conlon, G.; Fitzpatrick, P.; Daly, L. Gender and content influence second-level students' expectations of health education seminars provided in a health promoting hopital setting. *Clin. Health Promot.* **2014**, *4*, 5–11.
26. Hayes, S. A Critical Examination and Evaluation of the Place of Science in the Irish Transition Year. Ph.D. Thesis, University of Limerick, Limerick, Ireland, 2011.
27. Plotnikoff, R.C.; Costigan, S.A.; Karunamuni, N.; Lubans, D.R. Social cognitive theories used to explain physical activity behavior in adolescents: A systematic review and meta-analysis. *Prev. Med.* **2013**, *56*, 245–253. [CrossRef] [PubMed]
28. Davis, R.; Campbell, R.; Hildon, Z.; Hobbs, L.; Michie, S. Theories of behaviour and behaviour change across the social and behavioural sciences: A scoping review. *Health Psychol. Rev.* **2015**, *9*, 323–344. [CrossRef]
29. Bandura, A. Self-efficacy: Toward a unifying theory of behavioral change. *Psychol. Rev.* **1977**, *84*, 191–215. [CrossRef] [PubMed]
30. Martin, J.J.; Kulinna, P.H. A Social Cognitive Perspective of Physical-Activity-Related Behavior in Physical Education. *J. Teach. Phys. Educ.* **2005**, *24*, 265–281. [CrossRef]
31. Deci, E.L.; Ryan, R.M. *Intrinsic Motivation and Self-Determination in Human Behaviour*; Plenum Press: New York, NY, USA, 1985.
32. Hagger, M.S.; Chatzisarantis, N.L.D.; Culverhouse, T.; Biddle, S.J.H. The Processes by Which Perceived Autonomy Support in Physical Education Promotes Leisure-Time Physical Activity Intentions and Behavior: A Trans-Contextual Model. *J. Educ. Psychol.* **2003**, *95*, 784–795. [CrossRef]
33. Hagger, M.S.; Chatzisarantis, N.L.D.; Hein, V.; Soos, I.; Karsai, I.; Lintunen, T.; Leemans, S. Teacher, peer and parent autonomy support in physical education and leisure-time physical activity: A trans-contextual model of motivation in four nations. *Psychol. Health* **2009**, *24*, 689–711. [CrossRef] [PubMed]

34. Mameli, C.; Molinari, L.; Passini, S. Agency and responsibility in adolescent students: A challenge for the societies of tomorrow. *Br. J. Educ. Psychol.* **2019**, *89*, 41–56. [CrossRef]
35. McNeely, C.; Falci, C. School Connectedness and the Transition into and Out of Health-Risk Behavior Among Adolescents: A Comparison of Social Belonging and Teacher Support. *J. Sch. Health* **2004**, *74*, 284–292. [CrossRef]
36. Dowd, A.J.; Chen, M.Y.; Jung, M.E.; Beauchamp, M.R. "Go Girls!" psychological and behavioral outcomes associated with a group-based healthy lifestyle program for adolescent girls. *Transl. Behav. Med.* **2015**, *5*, 77–86. [CrossRef]
37. Prochaska, J.O.; DiClemente, C.C. Stages and processes of self-change of smoking: Toward an integrative model of change. *J. Consult. Clin. Psychol.* **1983**, *51*, 390–395. [CrossRef]
38. De Bourdeaudhuij, I.; Philippaerts, R.; Crombez, G.; Matton, L.; Wijndaele, K.; Balduck, A.; Lefevre, J. Stages of change for physical activity in a community sample of adolescents. *Health Educ. Res.* **2005**, *20*, 357–366. [CrossRef]
39. Eldridge, S.M.; Lancaster, G.A.; Campbell, M.J.; Thabane, L.; Hopewell, S.; Coleman, C.L.; Bond, C.M. Defining Feasibility and Pilot Studies in Preparation for Randomised Controlled Trials: Development of a Conceptual Framework. *PLoS ONE* **2016**, *11*, e0150205. [CrossRef]
40. Bowen, D.J.; Kreuter, M.; Spring, B.; Cofta-Woerpel, L.; Linnan, L.; Weiner, D.; Bakken, S.; Kaplan, C.P.; Squiers, L.; Fabrizio, C.; et al. How We Design Feasibility Studies. *Am. J. Prev. Med.* **2009**, *36*, 452–457. [CrossRef]
41. Thabane, L.; Ma, J.; Chu, R.; Cheng, J.; Ismaila, A.; Rios, L.P.; Robson, R.; Thabane, M.; Giangregorio, L.; Goldsmith, C.H. A tutorial on pilot studies: The what, why and how. *BMC Med. Res. Methodol.* **2010**, *10*, 1. [CrossRef]
42. Ferguson, C.J.; Heene, M. A Vast Graveyard of Undead Theories: Publication Bias and Psychological Science's Aversion to the Null. *Perspect. Psychol. Sci.* **2012**, *7*, 555–561. [CrossRef]
43. Rosenbaum, P.; Gorter, J.W. The 'F-words' in childhood disability: I swear this is how we should think! *Child Care Health Dev.* **2012**, *38*, 457–463. [CrossRef]
44. Ng, K.; Hämylä, R.; Tynjälä, J.; Villberg, J.; Tammelin, T.; Kannas, L.; Kokko, S. Test-retest reliability of adolescents' self-reported physical activity item in two consecutive surveys. *Arch. Public Health* **2019**, *77*, 9. [CrossRef] [PubMed]
45. Nigg, C.R.; Courneya, K.S. Transtheoretical model: Examining adolescent exercise behavior. *J. Adoles. Health* **1998**, *22*, 214–224. [CrossRef]
46. Prochaska, J.J.; Rodgers, M.W.; Sallis, J.F. Association of Parent and Peer Support with Adolescent Physical Activity. *Res. Q. Exerc. Sport* **2002**, *73*, 206–2010. [CrossRef] [PubMed]
47. Hagger, M.S.; Chatzisarantis, N.L.D.; Biddle, S.J.H. The influence of self-efficacy and past behaviour on the physical activity intentions of young people. *J. Sports Sci.* **2001**, *19*, 711–725. [CrossRef] [PubMed]
48. Lee, R.E.; Nigg, C.R.; Diclemente, C.C.; Courneya, K.S. Validating Motivational Readiness for Exercise Behavior with Adolescents. *Res. Q. Exerc. Sport* **2001**, *72*, 401–410. [CrossRef] [PubMed]
49. Felder-Puig, R.; Griebler, R.; Samdal, O.; King, M.A.; Freeman, J.G.; Duer, W. Does the School Performance Variable Used in the International Health Behavior in School-Aged Children (HBSC) Study Reflect Students' School Grades? *J. Sch. Health* **2012**, *82*, 404–409. [CrossRef] [PubMed]
50. Harter, S. The Perceived Competence Scale for Children. *Child Dev.* **1982**, *53*, 87–97. [CrossRef]
51. Ravens-Sieberer, U.; KIDSCREEN Group Europe. *The KIDSCREEN Questionnaires. Quality of Life Questionnaires for Children and Adolescents—Handbook*; Papst Science Publisher: Lengerich, Germany, 2006.
52. McKenzie, T.L.; Marshall, S.J.; Sallis, J.F.; Conway, T.L. Leisure-time physical activity in school environments: An observational study using SOPLAY. *Prev. Med.* **2000**, *30*, 70–77. [CrossRef]
53. Lancaster, G.A. Pilot and feasibility studies come of age! *Pilot Feasibility Stud.* **2015**, *1*, 1. [CrossRef] [PubMed]
54. Krueger, R.A. *Developing Questions for Focus Groups*; Sage: Thousand Oaks, CA, USA, 1998.
55. Vaughn, S.; Schumm, J.S.; Sinagub, J. *Focus Group Interviews in Education and Psychology*; Sage Research Methods: Thousand Oaks, CA, USA, 2018.
56. Hollander, J.A. The social contexts of focus groups. *J. Contemp Ethnogr.* **2004**, *33*, 602–637. [CrossRef]
57. McDonald, W.J.; Topper, G.E. Focus group research with children: A structural approach. *Appl. Mark. Res.* **1988**, *28*, 3–11.

58. Lederman, L.C. Assessing educational effectiveness: The focus group interview as a technique for data collection. *Commun. Educ.* **1990**, *39*, 117–127. [CrossRef]
59. Moran, A.P.; Matthews, J.J.; Kirby, K. Whatever happened to the third paradigm? Exploring mixed methods research designs in sport and exercise psychology. *Qual. Res. Sport Exerc. Health* **2011**, *3*, 362–369. [CrossRef]

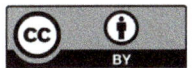

© 2019 by the authors. Licensee MDPI, Basel, Switzerland. This article is an open access article distributed under the terms and conditions of the Creative Commons Attribution (CC BY) license (http://creativecommons.org/licenses/by/4.0/).

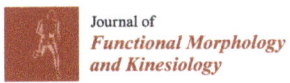

Brief Report

A 47-Year Comparison of Lower Body Muscular Power in Spanish Boys: A Short Report

Iván Chulvi-Medrano [1],*, Manuel Pombo [2], Miguel Ángel Saavedra-García [3], Tamara Rial Rebullido [4] and Avery D Faigenbaum [5]

[1] Sport Performance and Physical Fitness Research Group (UIRFIDE), Department of Physical and Sports Education, Faculty of Physical Activity and Sport Sciences, University of Valencia, 46010 Valencia, Spain
[2] Department of Physical Education and Sport, University of Coruña, 15179 A Coruña, Spain; pombo@udc.es
[3] Group of Research in Sport Science (INCIDE), Department of Physical Education and Sport, University of Coruña, 15179 A Coruña, Spain; miguel.saavedra@udc.es
[4] Exercise & Women's Health, Newtown, CT 18940, USA; rialtamara@gmail.com
[5] Department of Health and Exercise Science, The College of New Jersey, Ewing, NJ 08628, USA; faigenba@tcnj.edu
* Correspondence: ivan.chulvi@uv.es

Received: 11 July 2020; Accepted: 18 August 2020; Published: 20 August 2020

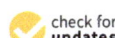

Abstract: Much of the evidence examining temporal trends in fitness among youth has found a decrease in measures of muscular strength and muscular power over recent decades. The aim of this study was to examine trends in lower body muscular power in Spanish boys over 47 years. In 1969 140 boys (10–11 years; body mass index = 19.24, SD = 2.91 kg/m^2) and in 2016, 113 boys (10–11 years; body mass index = 19.20, SD = 3.15 kg/m^2) were recruited. Lower body power was assessed using the vertical jump (VJ) and standing long jump (SLJ) tests. Significant differences and a large effect size were shown between groups in the SLJ ($p = 0.001$; d = 0.94) and the VJ ($p = 0.001$; d = 0.66). SLJ data in 1969 were higher (1.52 m, SD = 0.19) when compared to the 2016 data (1.34 m, SD = 0.18). The VJ performance of the 1969 sample was also higher (25.95 cm; SD = 6.58) than the 2016 sample (21.56 cm; SD = 4.72). SLJ and VJ performance of the 2016 group decreased 11.8% and 16.9%, respectively. There were no significant differences between groups in body mass index. The results indicate a secular decline in lower body muscular power in 10–11-year-old Spanish boys with no significant changes in body mass index over the 47-year study period.

Keywords: pediatric dynapenia; children; resistance training

1. Introduction

Low levels of muscular fitness (i.e., muscular strength, muscular power and local muscular endurance) in children and adolescents are associated with poor motor competence, functional limitations and adverse health outcomes [1,2]. Recent findings indicate that measures of muscular strength and power in modern-day youths are lower than in previous generations [3–6]. Sandercock and Cohen reported a decline in muscular fitness (bent-arm hang, sit-ups and handgrip) using allometric equations in 10-year-old English children from 1998 to 2014, and noted this trend was independent of secular changes in body size [5]. A similar trend in muscular fitness was observed in Spanish adolescents between 2001–2002 and 2006–2007 [4], and in an international sample of children and adolescents between 1964 and 2017 [7].

Lower levels of muscular strength and power in modern day youths appear to be consequent to lifestyles characterized by reduced physical activity and increased sedentary behavior [3,5,8]. Importantly, muscular strength and fundamental movement skill proficiency are considered foundational for ongoing participation in physical activity across the lifespan [8,9]. Therefore, it is critical to examine temporal trends in muscular fitness in youth due to the far-reaching implications for disease prevention and health promotion. A recent meta-analysis concluded that poor muscular fitness was associated with lower levels of bone mineral density and self-esteem, as well as higher levels of body fat and cardiometabolic risk [1]. In support of these observations, lower handgrip levels in youth with obesity have been associated with increased cardiometabolic risk [10]. Further, low levels of performance on selected measures of muscular fitness, including the handgrip, push-up and long jump early in life have been found to be associated with an increased risk of metabolic syndrome later in life [11]. Specifically, the long jump is a field test commonly used in youths as a general measure of lower body muscular fitness [12].

Temporal trends of muscular fitness performance in youth can be used to inform public health policies about youths' physical activity and health [13]. However, there are a limited number of studies examining trends in lower body muscular fitness in youths over recent decades. Additional data are needed to fill this research gap. The aim of this study was to describe temporal trends in lower body muscular power in Spanish boys over a 47-year time period from 1969 to 2016. We hypothesized that contemporary trends towards decreasing levels of muscular strength and muscular power shown in previous studies will be similar in Spanish children in 2016 as compared to Spanish children in 1969.

2. Materials and Methods

Data were collected from two separate cross-sectional samples from the same school in Galicia, Spain. The sample consisted of the total boys (10 to 11 years of age) enrolled in the school during both years. Participants included 140 boys (10–11 years; body mass index = 19.24, SD = 2.91 kg/m^2) in 1969 and 113 boys (10–11 years; body mass index = 19.20, SD = 3.15 kg/m^2) in 2016. The University Da Coruña Ethics Committee approved this research study and parents and participants were informed about experimental procedures and provided parental permission and child assent, respectively.

Body mass index (BMI) was calculated as body mass measured on an analogic scale to the nearest 0.1 kg divided by height measured on a stadiometer to the nearest 0.5 cm squared. Lower body power was assessed using the vertical jump (VJ) and standing long jump (SLJ) tests following standardized procedures [14]. In the SLJ the participant stood with both feet just behind the starting line on a marked floor. The distance between the starting line and the back edge of the participant's heel was measured after each jump. For the VJ test, participants were instructed to jump as high as possible and mark the wall with chalk on their fingers. The vertical jump was calculated by subtracting a participant's standing reach height from the maximal jump height. Participants were permitted to perform a countermovement prior to jumping vertically or horizontally. The test order was randomized, and all participants performed 3 trials per test. Participants were allowed to rest for 1 min between trials and for 3 min between the VJ and SLJ tests. The best score from each test was used for data analysis. In 2016, the same testing protocols and procedures were followed as in 1969. The VJ and SLJ were part of the Spanish physical education curricula during the study period and therefore all participants had 2 familiarization sessions with these tests.

A Kolmogorov–Smirnov test was conducted to determine whether the data met the assumptions of normality of distribution. When the data met the normal distribution, two-tailed t-tests were applied for normally distributed data and the Mann–Whitney test was used for non-normal data to determine differences between cohorts. Significance was stablished at $p < 0.05$. D-Cohen effect size (ES) was calculated using the recommended Equation (1) [15].

$$ES = \frac{\text{mean of the experimental group} - \text{mean of the control group}}{\text{standard deviation of the control group}} \quad (1)$$

3. Results

In 1969, the sample mean age was 10.53 (0.50) years-old (min 10- max 11-years-old) and the median was 11-years-old. In 2016, the sample mean age was 10.43 (0.49) years-old (min 10- max 11-years-old) and the median was 10-years-old. Characteristic outcomes in the different cohorts are presented in Table 1.

Table 1. Participant demographics and lower body muscle power over a 47-year-period in Spanish boys.

Variables	Sample 1 1969 n= 140 Mean (SD)	Sample 2 2016 n= 113 Mean (SD)	Δ	p-Value	Cohen's d
Height (cm)	147.06 (6.21)	140.25 (6.17)	−4.6	0.001	1.18
Mass (kg)	41.68 (6.21)	38.01(8.08)	−8.8	0.001	0.50
BMI [1] (kg/m^2)	19.24 (2.91)	19.20 (3.15)	−0.20%	0.473	0.01
SLJ [1] (m)	1.52 (0.19)	1.34 (0.8)	−11.8%	0.001	0.94
VJ [1] (vm)	25.95 (6.58)	21.56 (4.72)	−16.9%	0.001	0.66

[1] BMI: Body Mass Index; SLJ: Standing Long Jump; VJ: Vertical Jump.

4. Discussion

Significant differences and a large effect size were found in SLJ and VJ performance from 1969 to 2016. Over this 47-year period, SLJ performance decreased 11.8% and VJ decreased 16.9%. These results indicate a declining trend in lower body muscular power in 10–11-year-old Spanish boys with no significant changes in BMI. Our findings show a greater decline in SLJ than in previous research. We observed an 11.8% decline in SLJ between 1969 and 2016, whereas Moliner-Urdiales and colleagues found a decline in SLJ performance of 4.8% in 12.5- to 17.5-year-old Spanish adolescents assessed between 2001–2002 and 2006–2007 [4]. Similarly, Hardy and colleagues reported a decline in SLJ in youth between 1985 and 2015, with 10-year-old boys decreasing SLJ performance by 4.8% [13]. These trends in measures of lower body muscular strength and muscular power in youth may be explained by declining levels of regular participation in physical education, outdoor active play, and sport activities during the respective study periods [16]. Of interest, Tomkinson and colleagues quantified global changes in anaerobic fitness in more than 20 million youths and reported improvements in performance from 1958 to 1982, followed by a plateau and eventual decline in anaerobic test performance until 2003 [17]. This observed decline in anaerobic performance is consistent with our observed temporal trends in musculoskeletal fitness. Similarly, Kaster and colleagues evaluated temporal trends in sit-up performance in almost 10 million children and adolescents and reported large international improvements from 1964 to 2000 before then stabilizing near zero until 2010 before declining [7]. Of note, national trends in sit-up performance were strongly and positively associated with trends in vigorous physical activity, with countries with the largest improvements in sit-up performance reporting the largest increases in vigorous physical activity [7].

Another outcome of interest is the BMI. Our findings indicate that there was no significant difference in BMI between 1969 and 2016. However, the 2016 boys were shorter with a lower body mass than in 1969. These differences could be attributed to a younger age of development. While BMI in our study showed no significant differences over a 47-year period, other reports observed an increase in BMI over a period of 30 years [13]. Our findings are not consistent with others who reported that today's youths are taller and heavier than previous generations [13]. Of interest, the Spanish physical education curricula in the 1960s, 1970s and 1980s typically included more strength- and skill-building physical exercises, as compared to the more recent focus on aerobic games and activities. As such, trends in BMI and body composition must be viewed in light of the type and intensity of exercise performed, as well as the age, sex and biological maturation of the study participants.

We found a decrease in lower body power independent of changes in body size and BMI over the study period. The same downward trend in muscular fitness independent of secular changes in body size and BMI was also observed in 10-year-old English children, as reported by Sandercock and

Cohen [5]. While our 1969 sample was heavier and taller than our 2016 sample, with no significant differences in BMI, English children in the Sandercock and Cohen study were taller and heavier in 2014 than in 2008 and 1998, with no significant differences in BMI [5]. Collectively, these results suggest that changes in muscular fitness over time may not be associated with secular changes in BMI and body size. It is possible that other factors, such as trends in quality and quantity of physical activity engagement, may contribute to the observed decline in muscular fitness in modern day youths. This downward trend in muscular fitness in modern day youths has also been reported in children and adolescents from other countries [3]. It should be noted that, without regular opportunities to engage regularly in strength-building exercises, today's youths may be less likely to attain the adequate levels of muscular fitness that are needed for ongoing participation in MVPA [3,18]. Since low levels of muscular strength and power early in life are risk factors for pediatric dynapenia and associated health-related concerns [19], the SLJ has been suggested as a valid general index for assessing muscular fitness in youths [12].

Our results show that the 2016 cohort was shorter and their SLJ performance was significantly lower than in 1969. In young adults, SLJ performance has been found to be influenced by several factors, including anthropometrics [20]. Taller subjects have a higher center of gravity and longer leg lever that can produce greater mechanical jump forces. It has been reported that femur length has a significant influence on VJ performance [21]. In 10- to 12-year-old children, a positive moderate correlation between femur length and SJL, and a weak positive correlation between standing height and SLJ, were reported [22]. Given these observations, participant's anthropometrics may affect the take-off angle during the SLJ and, consequently, the jump distance.

Our study has several limitations that should be considered when interpreting the data. Notably, we included a relatively small sample of boys from Galicia, a region of Spain. Therefore, our data are not representative of all Spanish youths. Additionally, we did not assess the biologic maturation of the participants and we did not measure their current levels of physical activity with validated questionnaires. Additionally, we did not include the periodic testing of muscular fitness during the 47-year study period and, therefore, changes in performance during selected periods of time cannot be analyzed. The assessment of body composition in order to differentiate between lean body mass and fat mass was not performed. Additional research is warranted to address the changes in muscular phenotype (e.g., muscular strength and power) in girls and boys, while controlling for confounding variables, such as exercise participation and training history. Finally, it has been reported that sociodemographic variables [13] and the trends towards unhealthy eating habits [23] may influence fitness performance in youths; however, we did not assess these variables.

5. Conclusions

To the best of our knowledge no previous studies have examined temporal trends in muscular fitness in youths over a 47-year period. Our novel findings are consistent with other reports from western societies that highlight declines in measures of muscular strength and muscular power in modern day children and adolescents. To alter the current trajectory towards lower levels of muscular fitness in children and adolescents, developmentally appropriate interventions that target neuromuscular deficiencies and enhance muscular strength and power are needed to avert the troubling consequences of pediatric dynapenia.

Author Contributions: Conceptualization, M.P. and I.C.-M.; methodology, M.P. and M.Á.S.-G.; software, M.Á.S.-G.; formal analysis, I.C.-M., M.Á.S.-G., T.R.R., and A.D.F.; data curation, M.Á.S.-G, I.C.-M., T.R.R., and A.D.F.; writing—original draft preparation, I.C.-M., M.P., and M.Á.S.-G.; writing—review and editing, T.R.R. and A.D.F. All authors have read and agreed to the published version of the manuscript.

Funding: This research received no external funding.

Conflicts of Interest: The authors declare no conflict of interest.

References

1. Smith, J.J.; Eather, N.; Morgan, P.J.; Plotnikoff, R.C.; Faigenbaum, A.D.; Lubans, D.R. The health benefits of muscular fitness for children and adolescents: A systematic review and meta-analysis. *Sports Med.* **2014**, *44*, 1209–1223. [CrossRef] [PubMed]
2. García-Hermoso, A.; Ramírez-Campillo, R.; Izquierdo, M. Is muscular fitness associated with future health benefits in children and adolescents? A systematic review and meta-analysis of longitudinal studies. *Sports Med.* **2019**, *49*, 1079–1094. [CrossRef] [PubMed]
3. Faigenbaum, A.D.; Rebullido, T.R.; Peña, J.; Chulvi-Medrano, I. Resistance exercise for the prevention and treatment of pediatric dynapenia. *J. Sci. Sport Exerc.* **2019**, *1*, 208–216. [CrossRef]
4. Moliner-Urdiales, D.; Ruiz, J.R.; Ortega, F.B.; Jiménez-Pavón, D.; Vicente-Rodriguez, G.; Rey-López, J.P.; Martínez-Gómez, D.; Casajús, J.A.; Mesana, M.I.; Marcos, A.; et al. Secular trends in health-related physical fitness in Spanish adolescents: The AVENA and HELENA Studies. *J. Sci. Med. Sport* **2010**, *13*, 584–588. [CrossRef]
5. Sandercock, G.R.H.; Cohen, D.D. Temporal trends in muscular fitness of English 10-year-olds 1998–2014: An allometric approach. *J. Sci. Med. Sport* **2018**, *22*, 201–205. [CrossRef]
6. Cohen, D.; Voss, C.; Taylor, M.; Delextrat, A.; Ogunleye, A.; Sandercock, G. Ten-year secular changes in muscular fitness in English children. *Acta Paediatr. Int. J. Paediatr.* **2011**, *100*, 175–177. [CrossRef]
7. Kaster, T.; Dooley, F.L.; Fitzgerald, J.S.; Walch, T.J.; Annandale, M.; Ferrar, K.; Lang, J.J.; Smith, J.J.; Tomkinson, G.R. Temporal trends in the sit-ups performance of 9,939,289 children and adolescents between 1964 and 2017. *J. Sports Sci.* **2020**, 1–11. [CrossRef]
8. Smith, J.J.; Eather, N.; Weaver, R.G.; Riley, N.; Beets, M.W.; Lubans, D.R. Behavioral correlates of muscular fitness in children and adolescents: A systematic review. *Sport. Med.* **2019**, *49*, 887–904. [CrossRef]
9. Hulteen, R.M.; Morgan, P.J.; Barnett, L.M.; Stodden, D.F.; Lubans, D.R. Development of foundational movement skills: A conceptual model for physical activity across the lifespan. *Sport. Med.* **2018**, *48*, 1533–1540. [CrossRef]
10. Laitinen, T.T.; Saner, C.; Nuotio, J.; Sabin, M.A.; Fraser, B.J.; Harcourt, B.; Juonala, M.; Burgner, D.P.; Magnussen, C.G. Lower grip strength in youth with obesity identifies those with increased cardiometabolic risk. *Obes. Res. Clin. Pract.* **2020**, *14*, 286–289. [CrossRef]
11. Fraser, B.J.; Huynh, Q.L.; Schmidt, M.D.; Dwyer, T.; Venn, A.J.; Magnussen, C.G. Childhood muscular fitness phenotypes and adult metabolic syndrome. **2016**, *48*, 1715–1722. [CrossRef] [PubMed]
12. Castro-Piñero, J.; Ortega, F.B.; Artero, E.G.; Girela-Rejón, M.J.; Mora, J.; Sjöström, M.; Ruiz, J.R. Assessing muscular strength in youth: Usefulness of standing long jump as a general index of muscular fitness. *J. Strength Cond. Res.* **2010**, *24*, 1810–1817. [CrossRef] [PubMed]
13. Hardy, L.L.; Merom, D.; Thomas, M.; Peralta, L. 30-year changes in Australian children's standing broad jump: 1985–2015. *J. Sci. Med. Sport* **2018**, *21*, 1057–1061. [CrossRef]
14. Haff, G.G.; Tripplet, N. *Essentials of Strength Training and Conditioning*, 4th ed.; Human Kinetics Publishers Inc.: Champaing, IL, USA, 2016; pp. 267–269.
15. Rhea, M.R. Determining the magnitude of treatment effects in strength training research trough the use of the effect size. *J. Strength Cond. Res.* **2004**, *18*, 918–920. [CrossRef] [PubMed]
16. Aubert, S.; Barnes, J.D.; Abdeta, C.; Nader, P.A.; Adeniyi, A.F.; Aguilar-Farias, N.; Tenesaca, D.S.A.; Bhawra, J.; Brazo-Sayavera, J.; Cardon, G.; et al. Global Matrix 3.0 physical activity Report Card grades for children and youth: Results and analysis from 49 countries. *J. Phys. Act. Health* **2018**, *15*, S251–S273. [CrossRef]
17. Tomkinson, G.R. Global changes in anaerobic fitness test performance of children and adolescents (1958-2003). *Scand. J. Med. Sci. Sports* **2006**, *17*, 497–507. [CrossRef]
18. Stricker, P.R.; Faigenbaum, A.D.; Mccambridge, T.M.; Sports, O.N. Resistance training for children and adolescents. *Pediatrics* **2020**, *145*, e20201011. [CrossRef]
19. Faigenbaum, A.D.; MacDonald, J.P. Dynapenia: It's not just for grown-ups anymore. *Acta Paediatr.* **2017**, *106*, 696–697. [CrossRef]
20. Wakai, M.; Linthorne, N.P. Optimum take-off angle in the standing long jump. *Hum. Mov. Sci.* **2005**, *24*, 81–96. [CrossRef]
21. Sharma, H.B.; Gandhi, S.; Meitei, K.K.; Dvivedi, J.; Dvivedi, S. Anthropometric basis of vertical jump performance: A study in young Indian national players. *J. Clin. Diagn. Res.* **2017**, *11*, CC01–CC05. [CrossRef]

22. Sidhu, J.S. Physical attributes as indicator of performance for broad jumping. *Int. J. Curr. Res. Rev.* **2018**, *10*, 22–25. [CrossRef]
23. Ribas-Barba, L.; Serra-Majem, L.; Salvador, G.; Castell, C.; Cabezas, C.; Salleras, L.; Plasencia, A. Trends in dietary habits and food consumption in Catalonia, Spain (1992–2003). *Public Health Nutr.* **2007**, *10*, 1340–1353. [CrossRef] [PubMed]

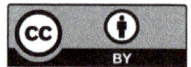

© 2020 by the authors. Licensee MDPI, Basel, Switzerland. This article is an open access article distributed under the terms and conditions of the Creative Commons Attribution (CC BY) license (http://creativecommons.org/licenses/by/4.0/).

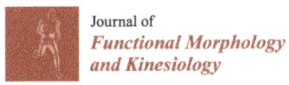 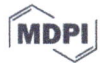

Review

Relation between Weight Status, Physical activity, Maturation, and Functional Movement in Adolescence: An Overview

Josip Karuc * and Marjeta Mišigoj-Duraković

Faculty of Kinesiology, University of Zagreb, Horvaćanski zavoj 15, 10 000 Zagreb, Croatia; marjeta.misigoj-durakovic@kif.hr
* Correspondence: josip.karuc@kif.hr; Tel.: +3859-1582-3504

Received: 4 April 2019; Accepted: 29 May 2019; Published: 30 May 2019

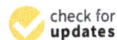

Abstract: Obesity, low level of physical activity and dysfunctional movement patterns presents one of the leading health issues that can contribute to increased risk for developing not only metabolic and cardiovascular disease, but also musculoskeletal problems. The aim of this paper is to summarize literature and evidence about relationship between functional movement (FM) patterns, physical activity (PA) level and weight status in average adolescent population. In addition, this paper summarized current evidence about relations between maturation effects and functional movement among athletic adolescent populations. Summary of current evidence suggests that decreased physical activity level is negatively correlated to functional movement in adolescence. Additionally, most studies suggest that weight status is negatively correlated to functional movement patterns although there is conflicting evidence in this area. Evidence consistently showed that overweight and obese adolescents exhibit poorer functional movement compared to normal weight adolescents. In addition, it appears that maturation has effects on functional movement in athletic populations of adolescents. It is therefore important that practitioners consider interventions which develop optimal functional movement alongside physical activity and weight management strategies in children, in order to reduce the risks of injuries and pathological abnormality arising from suboptimal movement patterns in later life.

Keywords: FMS; pubescence; pediatric population; fundamental movement

1. Introduction

According to WHO, obesity has tripled since 1975 and thus represents one of the leading world health problems [1]. Along with the obesity and overweight, low level of physical activity (PA) puts overweight children at a higher risk for developing noncommunicable diseases. Although PA level is important for health of the locomotor system and represents a quantitative measure of human movement, due to importance of locomotor health, qualitative aspects of movement need to be considered as well. Functional movement (FM) considers qualitative aspects of movement, and can be defined as optimal postural control and mobility of joints and body regions involved in a particular movement. On the other hand, dysfunctional movement patterns present low level of quality of FM and can be related to injury incidence and thus endanger musculoskeletal (MSK) health and can contribute to developing degenerative changes in adulthood.

Looking altogether, obesity, low level of PA, and dysfunctional movement, can contribute to even more increased risk for developing not only metabolic and cardiovascular disease, but also MSK problems in adulthood. Therefore, literature about mutual adverse effects of dysfunctional movement on mentioned variables need to be considered in order to provide practical information for professionals in the field of kinesiology, medicine, and related areas.

The importance and influence of PA and weight status on adolescent health has been investigated widely, however only few studies have examined the relationship between FM, PA level, and obesity among the pediatric population. To date, only few studies have examined FM in the general adolescent population [2–11]. There are only four studies that investigated relation between weight status and FM in children [8–11]. Additionally, only one study by Duncan and Stanley, investigated the association between FM and PA level among children [10]. However, no study appears to have summarized literature about functional movement and its relation to PA level, weight status, and maturation in the average adolescent population.

Therefore, the aim of this paper is to summarize literature and evidence about the relationship between FM patterns, PA level, and weight status in the average adolescent population. Additionally, this paper will summarize current evidence about relations between maturation effects and functional movement among the athletic adolescent population.

2. Materials and Methods

The author of this study conducted a search in PUBMED (from 1 January 1990 to 1 May 2019) searching for association between functional movement, weight status, physical activity level, and maturation in adolescent populations. Key words used for electronic searches were: "functional movement", "functional movement screen", "weight status", "physical activity", "physical activity level", and "maturation". Combining the key words "functional movement" and "functional movement screen" with the other key words: "adolescents", "intervention", "weight status", "physical activity", "physical activity level", and "maturation" were used according to Boolean logic. The studies were checked by one researcher (J.K.) and were searched by title/abstract. In this study, inclusion criteria were (1) studies that investigated functional movement on average adolescent population and exercise intervention aimed to improve functional movement outcomes in average adolescents, (2) studies that examined the association between functional movement and weight status and physical activity level in average adolescent populations, (3) studies that investigated the association between functional movement and maturation in athletic adolescent populations, and (4) English as a publication language. Exclusion criteria in this study were (1) studies that investigated adult populations, special populations (e.g., firefighters, officers, military population etc.) and populations with specific diseases or injuries, and (2) studies that investigated functional movement skills (FMS) or functional capacity/competence in pediatric populations were excluded as well. In addition, manually selected papers from references within selected researches were included in this paper.

3. Results

After an electronic search, the total number of studies that investigated functional movement via functional movement screen was 202. After inclusion and exclusion criteria were met, and after manually selection of references, 14 studies were included in this narrative review. After search, studies were categorized into three distinct areas: (1) functional movement in the average adolescent population and exercise intervention aimed to improve functional movement outcomes (six studies selected), (2) physical activity, weight status and functional movement among the adolescent population (four studies) and (3) maturation and functional movement among the athletic population of adolescents (four studies). Each of these study areas are incorporated and interpreted in the discussion section.

4. Discussion

4.1. Clinical Importance of the Functional Movement and Functional Movement Screen as a Diagnostic Tool

The Functional Movement Screen^{TM} (FMS^{TM}), originally created by Gray Cook and Lee Burton, is a screening instrument intended to evaluate deficiencies in mobility and stability [12,13]. FMS^{TM} includes seven tests: the deep squat, hurdle step, inline lunge, shoulder mobility, ASLR, trunk stability push-up and rotary stability. To the author's knowledge, this is the only diagnostic instrument available, described and validated in scientific literature for the purpose of screening functional movement patterns.

Scoring the FMS^{TM} has its own rules and procedures. The FMS raters use a standardized procedure to evaluate movement function. While performing FMS testing, each participant has a maximum of three trials for each test in accordance with the recommended protocol. Each test is scored on a three-point scale, from 0 to 3, with higher scores indicating better FM. In the presence of pain, a score of zero is noted. For each test, the highest score from three trials is recorded. An overall composite score was calculated with a total FMS score of 21 according to standardized guidelines. Descriptions of each FMS test, as well as standardized guidelines for the complete FMS testing is well written in the literature and can be studied elsewhere [12,13].

Some studies have shown the efficiency of the FMS in determining injury risk in athletes [14–16], however, others indicated the opposite [17–19]. Although there is conflicting evidence about the FMS as an injury predictive tool, the author's opinion is that the FMS has critical value for identifying movement mobility and stability deficiencies. Deficits in movement mobility and joint stability potentially predispose athletes and average populations to higher injury risk since optimal movement patterns can possibly prevent and reduce that risk.

Several studies reported moderate to good inter-rater and intra-rater reliability of the FMS even among novice raters [20,21]. In addition, two-hour education on using FMS as a diagnostic tool seems to be efficient according to prior research [21].

4.2. Functional Movement in the Average Adolescent Population and Exercise Intervention aimed to improve Functional Movement Outcomes

Although there are a number of studies that investigated functional movement among athletic adolescents, only few studies investigated FM in the average adolescent population. These studies investigated relations between FM and PA or weight status. Additionally, few studies investigated maturation effect on functional movement in the athletic adolescent population. Only one study provided normative values for the FMS in the adolescent population [2]. Another study investigated the prevalence of functional movement patterns in children over the first three years of post-primary education [3].

Abraham et al. [2] investigated functional movement patterns in the average population of adolescents. This study included a large number of participants ($n = 1005$) with ages from 10 to 17 years old. They reported a mean value of the total FMS score of 14.5 points. Additionally, results showed a significant difference in total FMS score between females and males. However, no significant difference in scores existed between those who reported a previous injury and those who did not. In addition, the authors suggested normative values for the individual functional movement patterns for this population that can be found in their paper [2]. However, there are few limitations of this study that should be considered while implementing normative values in the practice. Large age span (10–17 years) among participants in this study reveals that pre-pubertal and pubertal subjects were included in the sample. Additionally, this study excluded all inactive children which could potentially lead to higher mean values. Although there are few limitations in this study, this is the first study that provided normative values for a school aged adolescent population.

Lester et al. [3] examined the age-related association of functional movement among children in Ireland. The aim of this study was to gather data on prevalence of movement skills and functional movement patterns in children over the first three years of post-primary education ($n = 181$, mean age = 14.4). In this research, 43.6% of adolescents were in year one, 23.8% of adolescents were in year two and 32.6% adolescents were in year three with age range from 12.3 to 16.4 years old. Looking altogether, authors reported that results of the functional movement outcomes in their sample were suboptimal across all years. As authors stated, significant age-related differences were reported.

When we look this data, as age increases, scores on the in-line lunge pattern decrease (difference between the first and third year). Additionally, the mean total FMS score reported in this study was 14.05, which is similar to results obtained by Abraham et al. The authors of this study strongly suggest that school-based intervention should be incorporated across the post-primary education child population in order to decrease decline in the impaired movement patterns.

Four studies investigated the impact of exercise intervention on functional movement outcomes. Coker [4] investigated the impact of the standardized warm-up protocol in middle school children on functional movement parameters. Participants from seventh-grade and four eighth-grade physical education classes participated in this study ($n = 120$, mean age = 13.1 years old). A six-week intervention included exercises that targeted mobility and stability of joints and muscle activation (exercise targeted ankle joint mobility, pelvic stability and dysfunctional gluteal, abductors, and adductors muscles). Results of this study suggest that a warm-up, which consists of exercises that target typical movement and body dysfunctions among adolescents of a sensitive age, can significantly reduce dysfunctional movement patterns. It is the author's opinion that school policies should implement these programs into the physical education curriculum in order to reduce dysfunctional movement pattern prevalence and potentially reduce risk injury incidence among the average adolescent population.

A study done by Nourse et al. [5] investigated the impact of live video diet and exercise intervention on vascular and functional outcomes in overweight and obese children (mean age = 14.5, $n = 20$). The intervention lasted 12 weeks and included three times per week videoconferences with a trainer and diet consultations. Results of this study showed a significant reduction in waist-hip ratio and improvement in total functional movement screen score. Average improvement of the participants in total FMS score was 13 to 17 points, from baseline to the end of this intervention, respectively. Authors of study concluded that a 12-week live video intervention improves functional movement outcomes in the population of overweight and obese adolescents.

St Laurent et al. [6] investigated the impact of a suspension-training movement on functional movement in children ($n = 28$, average age = 9.3 years old). Participants were divided into two groups (control and intervention group). After the six-week suspension-training movement program was finished, the intervention group showed better results in functional movement outcomes relative to the control group. Authors of this study suggest that intervention using this kind of training modality could be beneficial for improving functional movement outcomes.

Wright et al. [7] examined the impact of fundamental movement training on functional movement outcomes in physically active children ($n = 22$, average age = 13.4). Participants were divided into two groups, where the intervention group was included in the training that focused on movement quality (weekly 4×30-min session) and participants from the control group were involved in multisport activity. Interestingly, results showed that short-term intervention focusing on movement quality did not have an effect on functional movement parameters in physically active children compared to the control group.

4.3. Physical Activity, Weight Status, and Functional Movement among Adolescent Populations

Although PA level and FM have critically important roles for general health of children, to date, only three studies appear to have examined relations between FM, weight status, and PA level among adolescents [8–11].

Study performed in Moldova investigated the relationship between FM, core strength, posture, and body mass index (BMI) [8]. Researchers collected data from 77 children, from 8 to 11 years old with an average BMI value of 16.4. Mitchell et al. reported the average total FMS score of 14.9 [8], which is slightly higher than the study done by Abraham et al. [2]. The results of this study showed that static posture and BMI are not related to FM. Additionally, researchers did not find a correlation between posture and FMS total score. These results are obvious since posture in this study was assessed in the static position while FMS tests assess movement and dynamic postural stabilization. On the other hand, results showed that core strength was positively related to the total FMS score. The authors of the study concluded that the individual test scores indicate that none of the test items were too difficult for the children, which means that the same tests can be directly used in clinical practice and school classes with school-aged children.

An interesting study done by Duncan et al. [9] examined the association between FM and overweight and obesity in British children. Data were obtained from 90 children, 7–10 years old. After BMI was determined, children were classified as normal weight, overweight, or obese according to international official guidelines. The results for total FMS score for normal weight children was 14.7, for overweight 12.2, and for obese children 9.0. Duncan et al., showed that total FMS score was negatively correlated with BMI. Additionally, the scores in all individual FMS tests were higher for normal weight children compared to obese children. In addition, normal weight children performed better than overweight children in the two tests: deep squat and shoulder mobility. On the other hand, overweight children scored better than obese children in four movement patterns (hurdle step, inline lunge, shoulder mobility, and ASLR). This result puts overweight and obese children in the group of children with increased risk for injury incidence. These are clinically important findings, because over time, dysfunctional movement patterns along with the effect of excess weight and consequently higher load on the joints, can possibly lead to degenerative changes in later life. This research highlights that overweight and obesity are significantly associated with poorer functional movement in children.

Findings of this study seems to be contradictory with the results of the study mentioned before [8]. However, in a study done by Mitchell et al., there are few limitations that need to be considered. The authors did not separate participants into three categories (normal weight, overweight, and obese). In addition, 9% of the children were categorized as overweight (with no information about number and percentage of obese children), whereas in study done by Duncan et al. one third of children were classified as overweight/obese [9]. This limitation can potentially lead to opposite results and limited conclusion, and therefore can minimize the importance of potential relations between higher values of the BMI and suboptimal functional movement patterns in children.

In this research field, one more interesting study was performed by the same authors [10]. Duncan and Stanley investigated relations between weight status, physical activity level, and functional movement in British children. This study was performed on 58, 10–11 year old children. The results showed that the total FMS score was negatively correlated with BMI and positively related to PA level. Normal weight children scored significantly better for total FMS score compared to children classified as overweight/obese. The mean of total FMS scores was 15.5 for normal weight children and 10.6 in overweight/obese children.

Duncan and Stanley explained these results through few possible mechanisms. These authors suggested that deficits in FM could exist prior to being overweight. They pointed out that: "Excess weight and functional prowess are the results of natural selection since children who are functionally limited will remain inactive and will not develop optimal functional movement patterns that underpin performance to the same level of mastery as children without functional limitation." [10]. Additionally, the authors discussed that children who are not functionally limited may more likely enjoy PA, and thus, engage in more regular practice of functional movement patterns that underpin performance. Looking altogether, the results presented in these studies support the need for interventions to increase level of physical activity and improve functional movement in overweight and obese pediatric populations.

Garcia-Pinillos et al. [11] examined relations between functional movement patterns and weight status in children aged between 6 and 13 years old ($n = 333$). Results of this study show that weight status is moderately negatively correlated with total FMS score. In addition, overweight and obese children showed poorer functional movement compared to normal weight children. These results are consistent with the study done by Duncan et al. In addition, significant differences were found between normal weight, overweight, and obese children in lower-extremity movement patterns (deep squat, hurdle step, in-line lunge) and flexibility tests (shoulder mobility, straight leg-raise), but also in trunk stability pattern (push-up). This research revealed that girls outperformed boys in tests that require flexibility and balance, while boys outperformed girls in stability tests which support previous findings in context of sex dimorphism in individual functional movement patterns [2].

The information presented in the paragraphs above are essentially important for the practice of physical education teachers, coaches, and other professionals who work with pediatric populations. Optimal level of PA and optimal FM in children can reduce the risks of orthopedic abnormality arising from suboptimal movement patterns in later life. Since suboptimal movement patterns and low PA level could predispose children to a higher risk of the injury incidence, practitioners should consider functional movement interventions. It is the author's opinion that this population needs specific exercises that address suboptimal movement patterns first, and then exercises targeting weight status to minimize risk of high-load exercise on the skeletal system in the pediatric population.

4.4. Maturation and Functional Movement among Athletic Populations of Adolescents

To date, a number of studies investigated maturation effects in the average and athletic population of adolescents. However, only few studies appear to have examined the relationship between maturity and functional movement patterns [22–25]. These studies included only the athletic adolescent population. Within this paragraph, the author will briefly provide a review of current evidence and conclusions about maturation effects on functional movement among athletic adolescents.

A study done by Portas et al. investigated the effect of maturity on functional movement screen scores in elite, adolescent soccer players [22]. The authors showed that maturity has substantial effects on FMS performance. Although this research highlights that findings are relevant only to those analyzing movement of soccer players, the authors of the mentioned study concluded that FMS assessment appears to be invalid for practical usage for very young players.

Paszkewicz et al. compared functional and static evaluation tools among adolescent athletes [23]. The authors of this study compared FMS scores and Beighton and Horan joint mobility index (BHJMI) scores among pubescence in adolescent athletes. Based on the results of the modified pubertal maturation observational scale, the authors separated subjects into three groups: prepubescent, early-pubescent, and postpubescent groups. The researchers revealed a main effect for FMS scores across pubertal groups, but not in BHJMI composite scores. The postpubescent participants had higher FMS scores compared with the prepubescent participants and the early-pubescent athletes. Additionally, the results of this study did not confirm any correlation between FMS composite scores and BHJMI composite scores. The results of this study suggest that the FMS can discriminate between levels of pubescence and detect alterations during the pubertal growth cycle, whereas the BHJMI may not.

Lloyd et al. examined relationships between functional movement screen scores, maturation, and physical performance in young soccer players [24]. This study demonstrated that variation of physical performance of youth soccer players could be explained by a combination of both functional movement screen scores and maturation.

Wright and Chesterton [25] aimed to investigate differences between individual functional movement patterns at different stages of maturation in young athletes (mean age = 14.1 years, age between 8 and 18 years old) from various sports (field athletics, endurance sport, team sports, combat, and water sports). Participants were categorized in the three distinct maturation groups, participants who were before, at, and after their adolescent growth spurt (peak height velocity (PHV)). The authors found that differences among these groups were greatest in movement patterns that have high demands on stability, which suggests that adolescents potentially develop stability in this period of growth. These findings are consistent with studies mentioned before in this section [22,23]. In addition, results of the push-up test were higher in children who were at growth spurt or after growth spurt, when compared with children before growth spurt. In addition, authors of this study concluded that maturation has no effect on total FMS score.

However, it appears that there is no study that investigated the relationship between maturation effects and functional movement patterns among the average adolescent population. Due to the importance of this research field, the author is of the opinion that more studies are necessary in this research field.

5. Conclusions

This paper gave a detailed description and summarization of the current literature in the field of pediatric PA level, obesity, and maturation related to functional movement. Although there are only few studies in this field of research, the author highlights the importance and health benefits of optimal FM in children, as well as the consequences of dysfunctional movement patterns on the health of the locomotor system. Summary of current evidence suggests that decreased physical activity level is negatively correlated to functional movement in adolescence. Additionally, most studies suggest that weight status is negatively correlated to functional movement patterns, although there is conflicting evidence in this area. Evidence consistently showed that overweight and obese adolescent exhibit poorer functional movement compared to normal weight adolescents. Most of the studies that examined effects of exercise intervention on functional movement improved functional movement outcomes, while one study showed the opposite. It is clear that more research is needed on this topic to establish true intervention effects. In addition, it appears that maturation has effects on functional movement in the athletic population of adolescents. It is therefore important that practitioners consider interventions which develop optimal functional movement alongside physical activity and weight management strategies in children, in order to reduce the risks of injuries and pathological abnormality arising from suboptimal movement patterns in later life.

Funding: This work was funded by the Croatian Science Foundation, foundation under the number IP-06-2016-9926 and DOK-2018-01-2328.

Conflicts of Interest: The authors declare no conflict of interest.

References

1. World Health Organization. WHO Media Centre. Obesity and overweight: Fact sheet. Available online: www.who.int/mediacentre/factsheets/fs311/en/ (accessed on 29 May 2019).
2. Abraham, A.; Sannasi, R.; Nair, R. Normative values for the functional movement screentm in adolescent school aged children. *Int. J. Sports Phys. Ther.* **2015**, *10*, 29–36.
3. Lester, D.; McGrane, B.; Belton, S.; Duncan, M.J.; Chambers, F.C.; O' Brien, W. The Age-Related Association of Movement in Irish Adolescent Youth. *Sports* **2017**, *5*, 77. [CrossRef] [PubMed]
4. Coker, C.A. Improving Functional Movement Proficiency in Middle School Physical Education. *Res. Q. Exerc. Sport* **2018**, *89*, 367–372. [CrossRef]
5. Nourse, S.E.; Olson, I.; Popat, R.A.; Stauffer, K.J.; Vu, C.N.; Berry, S.; Kazmucha, J.; Ogareva, O.; Couch, S.C.; Urbina, E.M.; et al. Live Video Diet and Exercise Intervention in Overweight and Obese Youth: Adherence and Cardiovascular Health. *J. Pediatr.* **2015**, *167*, 533–539.e1. [CrossRef] [PubMed]
6. St Laurent, C.W.; Masteller, B.; Sirard, J. Effect of a Suspension-Trainer-Based Movement Program on Measures of Fitness and Functional Movement in Children: A Pilot Study. *Pediatr. Exerc. Sci.* **2018**, *30*, 364–375. [CrossRef]
7. Wright, M.D.; Portas, M.D.; Evans, V.J.; Weston, M. The effectiveness of 4 weeks of fundamental movement training on functional movement screenand physiological performance in physically active children. *J. Strength. Cond. Res.* **2015**, *29*, 254–261. [CrossRef] [PubMed]
8. Mitchell, U.H.; Johnson, A.W.; Adamson, B. Relationship between functional movement screen scores, core strength, posture, and body mass index in school children in moldova. *J. Strength. Cond. Res.* **2015**, *29*, 1172–1179. [CrossRef]
9. Duncan, M.J.; Stanley, M.; Leddington Wright, S. The association between functional movement and overweight and obesity in British primary school children. *Sport Med. Arthrosc. Rehabil. Ther. Technol.* **2013**, *5*, 11. [CrossRef] [PubMed]
10. Duncan, M.J.; Stanley, M. Functional movement is negatively associated with weight status and positively associated with physical activity in British primary school children. *J. Obes.* **2012**, *2012*. [CrossRef] [PubMed]

11. García-Pinillos, F.; Roche-Seruendo, L.E.; Delgado-Floody, P.; Jerez Mayorga, D.; Latorre-Román, P.Á. Is there any relationship between functional movement and weight status? A study in Spanish school-age children. *Nutr. Hosp.* **2018**, *35*, 805–810.
12. Cook, G.; Burton, L.; Hoogenboom, B. Pre-Participation Screening: The Use of Fundamental Movements As An Assessment of Function–Part 1. *North Am. J. Sport Phys. Ther.* **2006**, *1*, 62–72.
13. Cook, G.; Burton, L.; Hoogenboom, B. Pre-Participation Screening: The Use of Fundamental Movements As An Assessment of Function–Part 2. *North Am. J. Sport Phys. Ther.* **2006**, *1*, 132–139.
14. Kiesel, K.B.; Butler, R.J.; Plisky, P.J. Prediction of Injury by Limited and Asymmetrical Fundamental Movement Patterns in American Football Players. *J. Sport Rehabil.* **2014**, *23*, 88–94. [CrossRef]
15. Garrison, M.; Westrick, R.; Johnson, M.R.; Benenson, J. Association between the functional movement screen and injury development in college athletes. *Int. J. Sports Phys. Ther.* **2015**, *10*, 21–28. [PubMed]
16. Shojaedin, S.S.; Letafatkar, A.; Hadadnezhad, M.; Dehkhoda, M.R. Relationship between functional movement screening score and history of injury and identifying the predictive value of the FMS for injury. *Int. J. Inj. Contr. Saf. Promot.* **2014**, *21*, 355–360. [CrossRef]
17. Dossa, K.; Cashman, G.; Howitt, S.; West, B.; Murray, N. Can injury in major junior hockey players be predicted by a pre-season functional movement screen—A prospective cohort study. *J. Can. Chiropr. Assoc.* **2014**, *58*, 421–427.
18. Bardenett, S.M.; Micca, J.J.; DeNoyelles, J.T.; Miller, S.D.; Jenk, D.T.; Brooks, G.S. Functional Movement Screen Normative Values and Validity in High School Athletes: Can the Fms™ Be Used As a Predictor of Injury? *Int. J. Sports Phys. Ther.* **2015**, *10*, 303–308. [PubMed]
19. Dorrel, B.S.; Long, T.; Shaffer, S.; Myer, G.D. Evaluation of the Functional Movement Screen as an Injury Prediction Tool Among Active Adult Populations: A Systematic Review and Meta-analysis. *Sports Health* **2015**, *7*, 532–537. [CrossRef]
20. Teyhen, D.S.; Shaffer, S.W.; Lorenson, C.L.; Halfpap, J.P.; Donofry, D.F.; Walker, M.J.; Dugan, J.L.; Childs, J.D. The Functional Movement Screen: A Reliability Study. *J. Orthop. Sport Phys. Ther.* **2012**, *42*, 530–540. [CrossRef]
21. Smith, C.A.; Chimera, N.J.; Wright, N.J.; Warren, M. Interrater and intrarater reliability of the functional movement screen. *J. Strength. Cond. Res.* **2013**, *27*, 982–987. [CrossRef] [PubMed]
22. Portas, M.D.; Parkin, G.; Roberts, J.; Batterham, A.M. Maturational effect on Functional Movement Screen™ score in adolescent soccer players. *J. Sci. Med. Sport* **2016**, *19*, 854–858. [CrossRef]
23. Paszkewicz, J.R.; McCarty, C.W.; Van Lunen, B.L. Comparison of Functional and Static Evaluation Tools Among Adoslecent Athletes. *J. Strength. Cond. Res.* **2013**, *27*, 2842–2850. [CrossRef] [PubMed]
24. Lloyd, R.S.; Oliver, J.L.; Radnor, J.M.; Rhodes, B.C.; Faigenbaum, A.D.; Myer, G.D. Relationships between functional movement screen scores, maturation and physical performance in young soccer players. *J. Sports Sci.* **2015**, *33*, 11–19. [CrossRef]
25. Wright, M.D.; Chesterton, P. Functional Movement Screen™ total score does not present a gestalt measure of movement quality in youth athletes. *J. Sports Sci.* **2019**, *37*, 1393–1402. [CrossRef] [PubMed]

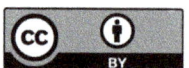

© 2019 by the authors. Licensee MDPI, Basel, Switzerland. This article is an open access article distributed under the terms and conditions of the Creative Commons Attribution (CC BY) license (http://creativecommons.org/licenses/by/4.0/).

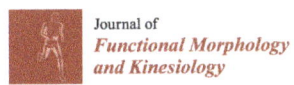

Review

The Effects of Alcohol Consumption on Recovery Following Resistance Exercise: A Systematic Review

Nemanja Lakićević

Sport and Exercise Research Unit, Department of Psychological, Pedagogical and Educational Sciences, University of Palermo, 90144 Palermo, Italy; nemanja.lakicevic@unipa.it; Tel.: +39-3515881179

Received: 14 May 2019; Accepted: 21 June 2019; Published: 26 June 2019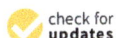

Abstract: Background: The aim of this manuscript was to describe the effects of alcohol ingestion on recovery following resistance exercise. Methods: A literature search was performed using the following database: Web of Science, NLM Pubmed, and Scopus. Studies regarding alcohol consumption after resistance exercise evaluating recovery were considered for investigation. The main outcomes took into account biological, physical and cognitive measures. Multiple trained researchers independently screened eligible studies according to the eligibility criteria, extracted data and assessed risk of bias. Results: A total of 12 studies were considered eligible and included in the quantitative synthesis: 10 included at least one measure of biological function, 10 included at least one measure of physical function and one included measures of cognitive function. Conclusions: Alcohol consumption following resistance exercise doesn't seem to be a modulating factor for creatine kinase, heart rate, lactate, blood glucose, estradiol, sexual hormone binding globulin, leukocytes and cytokines, C-reactive protein and calcium. Force, power, muscular endurance, soreness and rate of perceived exertion are also unmodified following alcohol consumption during recovery. Cortisol levels seemed to be increased while testosterone, plasma amino acids, and rates of muscle protein synthesis decreased.

Keywords: strength; training; muscle mass; muscle function; performance

1. Introduction

Resistance exercise (RE) is a commonly practiced modality of physical exercise used by both amateurs and elite athletes [1]. RE is a type of exercise that has gained a lot of interest over the past two decades, specifically for its role in improving athletic performance by developing muscular strength, power and speed, hypertrophy, local muscular endurance, motor performance, balance, and coordination [2]. While non-athletes use it to simply develop muscular physique, professional athletes engage in RE to enhance their athletic capabilities in various sports [3]. Variables such as exercise intensity, exercise frequency, load, number of sets and repetitions, rest periods and training volume can be manipulated in order to maximize RE induced effects in terms of muscle hypertrophy and strength [4]. Physiological and psychological constraints leading to a reduction in physical or mental performance can be classified as fatigue which is a phenomenon that has protective role in human physiology [5]. Exercise is a potent stimulus with respect to altering homeostatic variables which triggers adaptive reactions that counter the metabolic changes and repair the structural damage caused by the previous training session [5]. The stressful effects of RE can temporarily impair athlete's performance [6]. Therefore, the speed and quality of recovery are absolutely essential for the high performance athlete and, if done correctly, optimal recovery can lead to numerous benefits training and upcoming competition [7]. The main purpose of recovery is to restore physiological and psychological processes, so that the person engaging in vigorous exercise can repeat training sessions at an appropriate level [7]. It is also typically dependent on the nature of the exercise performed and any other outside stressors that the athlete may be exposed to [7].

Certainly, one of the unnecessary stressors during recovery phase is alcohol (ALC) consumption [8,9]. Worldwide, alcohol is the most commonly used psychoactive drug; it is estimated that each adult person consumes, on average, about 4.3 L of pure alcohol per year [10]. In the current era, consumption of alcohol is increasing exponentially in Western society [11–13] and it is common knowledge that alcohol can permeate virtually every organ and tissue in the body, resulting in tissue injury and organ dysfunction [14]. Alcohol consumption results in hormonal disturbances that can disrupt the physiological ability to maintain homeostasis and eventually can lead to various disorders, such as cardiovascular diseases, reproductive deficits, immune dysfunction, certain cancers, bone disease, and psychological and behavioral disorders [14]. In terms of post exercise recovery, acute alcohol ingestion reduces muscle protein synthesis in a dose-and time-dependent manner, after the cessation of exercise stimulus [8]. Alcohol does this mainly by suppressing the phosphorylation and activation of the mTOR pathways, the crucial kinase cascade regulating translation initiation [8,15]. Concomitantly, alcohol increases the expression of muscle specific enzymes that are up regulated by conditions that promote skeletal muscle atrophy [8,16].

Emerging research provides new insights into the effect of alcohol consumption on post-exercise muscle recovery but more research is needed to determine how this relationship exists and establish the physiological mechanisms governing this response. Therefore, the aim of this review is to understand the effects of alcohol consumption during recovery, on muscle function, following RE.

2. Materials and Methods

Preferred Reporting Items for Systematic Reviews and Meta-Analyses (PRISMA) statement has been used to structure this manuscript.

2.1. Inclusion and Exclusion Criteria

Studies that meet the following criteria will be included or excluded in this systematic review.

2.2. Eligibility Criteria

When it comes to eligibility criteria, only articles written in English language and published in peer-reviewed journals have been considered during the search. There was no limit on publication date when it comes to article eligibility. Different formats of publications such as reviews, meta-analysis, abstracts, citations, scientific conference abstracts, opinion pieces, books, book reviews, statements, letters, editorials, non-peer reviewed journal articles and commentaries have been excluded. With respect to intervention, publications were included only if they used a specific measure of performance or biomarker, that considered recovery following RE and alcohol intoxication. Articles exploring recovery after endurance type of training have been eliminated.

2.3. Participants

All the analyzed participants were adults to whom an ALC intervention was administered following a bout of RE. Children were not considered for analysis. There was no limitation when it comes to age, gender, number of participants, and duration of intervention or follow up period. Furthermore, there was no limitation when it comes to training status.

2.4. Interventions

The interventions described in the eligibility criteria will be included in this review. The interventions aimed to understand the effects of ALC on biological, physical and cognitive measures following RE. According to the nature of the review different methodological approaches which evaluate similar outcomes will be considered.

2.5. Comparators

Comparators will be control groups (people not consuming ALC [NO-ALC]) if present or if cross-over designs will be adopted the intervention groups will act as controls after each wash-out period.

2.6. Outcomes

The primary outcome will be to understand the effects of ALC compared to the NO-ALC intervention. Such findings will be applied to all the biological, physical and cognitive measures retrieved.

2.7. Search Strategy

We used EndNote v. 8.1 software (Clarivate Analytics, Jersey, UK) for the article search. The papers have been collected through PubMed (NLM), Web of Science (TS), and Scopus using the string: ((("alcohol" AND "exercise*" and "recovery*"; "ethanol" AND "exercise" AND "recovery"; "alcohol*" AND "resistance training" AND "recovery"; "ethanol" AND "resistance training*" AND "recovery"; "alcohol*" AND "strength*" AND "recovery"; "ethanol" AND "strength" AND "recovery"; "alcohol*" AND "training" AND "recovery"; "ethanol" and "training" and "recovery")).

2.8. Selection of Study Objects

The article screening was carried out in a three-step process: title reading, abstract reading and full text reading, respectively. If any disagreements were noticed between the two investigators, a third one considered the current process independently and discussed the decision with the other investigators. Furthermore, investigators were not blinded to the manuscripts, study title, authors, or associated institutions during the selection process. Both qualitative and quantitative articles were included in the review. The screening processes have been summarized via PRISMA flow diagram (Figure 1).

2.9. Risk of Bias

Risk of bias for the included studies was assessed through Downs and Black checklist [17]. This tool is useful when evaluating the quality of original research articles in order to synthesize evidence for public health purposes. This checklist contains 27 'yes'-or-'no' questions over five different domains. It offers both an overall score for study quality and a numeric score out of a possible 32 points. The five domains contain questions about study quality, external validity, study bias, confounding and selection bias, and power of the study.

Two independent researchers have completed the Downs and Black checklist of all included articles to determine the quality of each study. The maximum score a study can receive is 32, with higher scores indicating better quality. The studies were then divided into groups and marked as 'high quality' (score 23–32), 'moderate quality' (score 19–22), 'lower quality' (score 16–18) or 'poor quality' (<14) (Supplementary File S1 and S2). Kendall Tau correlation coefficient statistical method was used to determine inter-rater reliability. We used R statistical software (Bell Laboratories, Murray Hill, NJ, USA) version 3.6 to perform this analysis. Quality of evidence was determined by the study design and by Downs and Black score.

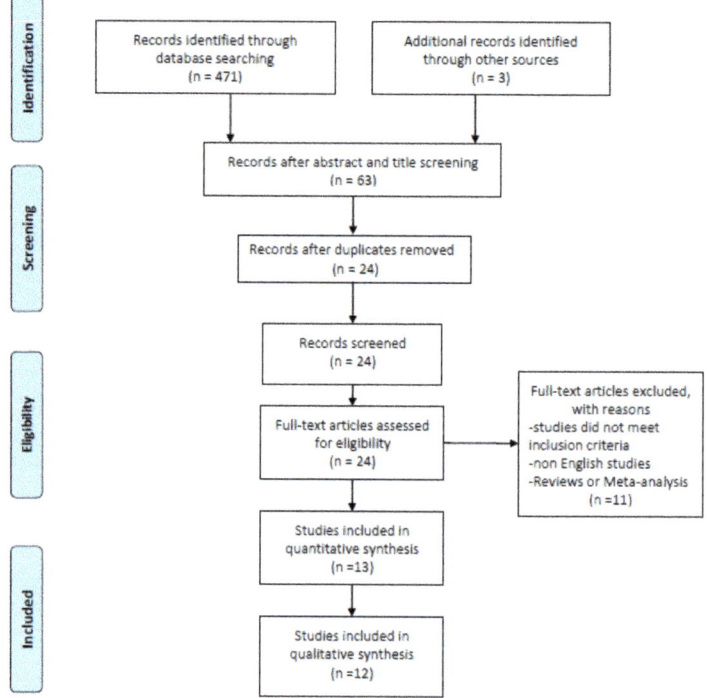

Figure 1. Prisma Flow Diagram

2.10. Data Synthesis

The critical information acquired from the included articles was extracted into Microsoft Excel for Macintosh, version 14.0 (Microsoft Corp, Redmond, WA, USA) spreadsheet. The most important characteristics of the studies, as author name and publication year, sample size, aim, alcohol dose, how this was mixed and administered, the study measures, the RE protocol adopted, the study design and the outcomes have been delineated in the tables while certain specifics about the particular study were described in a narrative manner.

3. Results

From a preliminary title and abstract search, a total number of 471 studies have been identified in the three screened databases. After the application of inclusion criteria on each article's title and abstract, 63 records were considered eligible. Duplicates were removed leaving 24 studies for full text screening. After full text screening, two additional studies from the relevant bibliography have been added. Of the 24 studies analyzed, 10 were included for the final synthesis. Therefore a total number of 12 studies were included in the qualitative synthesis of this review article. The process of article inclusion has been synthesized in Figure 1. Risk of bias assessment was finalized through Downs and Black checklist for all included studies (Supplementary File S1 and S2). The mean score was 19 (range = 12–28). After performing the inter-rater reliability test via Kendall Tau analysis we detected the score of 0.46 which can be classified as moderate but significant (p-value 0.026). As previously stated, after comprehensive screening, files were split into different quality categories in accordance to predetermined quality criteria (Supplementary File S1 and S2).

In order to evaluate the effects of alcohol consumption on recovery following RE, the results have been summarized into three categories: (1) biological and (2) physical measures and (3) cognitive function.

Of the retrieved studies, 10 took into account at least one biological measure [9,18–26], 11 took into account at least one physical measure [9,18–25,27,28] and cognitive function only one [24].

The retrieved biological measures include creatine kinase (CK) [18–25], heart rate [19,26], lactate [19,26], blood glucose [9], urine measures [24], cortisol [19,21,24,26], testosterone [19,21,24,26], estradiol [26], sexual hormone binding globulin (SHBG) [21,26], leukocytes and cytokines [19,21,22], C-reactive protein (CRP) [24], plasma amino acids [9], intracellular signaling proteins and rates of muscle protein synthesis (MPS) [9] and calcium (Ca^{2+}) [25]. The physical measures include force [18,20–25,27,28], power [19,21,24,28], muscular endurance [25], soreness [18,20,22,23,28] and rate of perceived exertion (RPE) [19,24,26]. The cognitive measures included a modified version of the STROOP test which evaluated time and accuracy of each response for congruent and incongruent stimuli. The alcohol dose provided to the participants in the included studies ranged between 0.6g/kg to 1.5g/kg. As defined by Kalinowski and Humphreys [29] a standard drink equals to 10 g of alcohol. Therefore, the alcohol dose provided to the participants, if we consider a man of 70kg, equals to 42 to 105 g of alcohol (4.2 to 10.5 standard drinks), which corresponds to 3 bottles of beer of 330 mL at 5% alcohol or a 370mL bottle of spirit at 37.5% alcohol, respectively. All the included studies adopted a cross-over research design. A summary of the retrieved studies is shown in Table 1.

3.1. Biological Measures

3.1.1. Creatine Kinase

Eight studies included CK measurement [18–25]. All the retrieved studies showed that CK increases following each RE protocol in both ALC and NO-ALC conditions showing a time interaction with RE. However, when analysing interaction with the different conditions, no differences were shown between the ALC and NO-ALC condition for none of the retrieved studies. Clarkson et al. [20], have also correlated peak CK activity from the ALC and the NO-ALC condition and found a high correlation coefficient ($r=0.95$), whereas Paulsen et al. [25] have also stratified the findings for man and women finding again no differences between the two groups neither for time or treatment assessment. Such results, as also highlighted by each author of the included studies, demonstrate that ALC cannot be considered as a modulating factor for CK following RE and that the increases of CK are the result of muscle damage following the exercise bouts.

3.1.2. Heart Rate

Two studies included measures of heart rate [19,26]. In both studies heart rate increased following the exercise intervention, however no difference was shown between the ALC and the NO-ALC condition.

3.1.3. Lactate

Two studies included measures of lactate [19,26]. In both studies lactate increased following the exercise intervention, however no difference was shown between the ALC and the NO-ALC condition.

3.1.4. Blood glucose

Only Parr et al. [9] evaluated the concentration of blood glucose. It has to be noted that Parr administered a concentration of alcohol in conjunction with either CHO or PRO. The results highlight a significant time and treatment interaction. Blood glucose concentration increased 0.5 and 4.5 h post intervention in the ALC-CHO group but not in the ALC-PRO or NO-ALC groups. Such findings demonstrate that blood glucose is affected by CHO but not ALC during recovery after RE.

Table 1. Descriptive characteristics of the retrieved studies.

Author [Ref] (Year)	n	Aim	Alcohol (dose)	Mix	Administration Time	Measures	Resistance Training	Comparator	Outcomes (Compared to Comparator)
Barnes et al. [27] (2010)	12	Evaluate if ALC interacts with damaged muscles.	1g/kg	37.5% ALC/volume; Smirnoff Vodka in orange juice (ratio 3.2:1)	A beverage was consumed every 15 min over a total time of 90 min.	-Strength. -Peak and averaged torque.	300 maximal eccentric contractions of the quadriceps muscles of one lower limb at an angular speed of 30°/s.	Cross-Over	No differences in acute performance measures. Decreased performance was seen after 36h following ingestion.
Barnes et al. [18] (2010)	11	To compare the effects of post-exercise ALC ingestion with that of an isocaloricnon-ALC beverage on changes in muscle performance.	1g/kg	37.5% ALC/volume; Smirnoff Vodka in orange juice (ratio 3.2:1).	A beverage was consumed every 15 min over a total time of 90 min.	-Soreness -Peak and averaged torque -CK	300 maximal eccentric contractions of the quadriceps muscles of one lower limb at an angular speed of 30°/s.	Cross-Over	Peak concentric, eccentric were lower in the ALC group. No differences in CK and soreness
Barnes et al. [19] (2012)	10	To investigate the effects of post-game ALC consumption on whole-body, sport-specific performance.	1g/kg	37.5% ALC/volume; Smirnoff Vodka in orange juice (ratio 3.2:1).	A beverage was consumed every 15 min over a total time of 90 min.	-HR -Lactate -RPE -CMJ -HPO -CK -Cortisol and Testosterone -Leukocytes	BURST Protocol (intense 20-m shuttle run with 180° turns)	Cross-Over	HR and Lactate showed no difference. RPE varied significantly. Differences in CMJ but not in HPO were present. No differences in the leukocyte count. CK was higher in the ALC group only after 48h. Testosterone did not show any differences. Cortisol was higher in the ALC group after 36h.
Clarkson et al. [20] (1990)	10	Assess the effect of acute ALC ingestion on muscle indicators.	0.8g/kg	Vodka 40% with orange juice (ratio 1:1)	Single dose.	-CK -Soreness -Isometric strength	50 repetitions at a lat-pulley.	Cross-Over.	No difference in CK. No difference in soreness. No difference in strength.
Haugvad et al. [21] (2014)	9	Investigate the effects of ethanol on recovery of muscle function after RT.	-Low dose 0.6 or 0.7 g/kg -High dose 1.2 or 1.4 g/kg	40% ethanol/volume; Absolut vodka diluted with 200-mL sugar-free lemonade(raspberry flavour) and water to a total of 1.5 L.	The beverage was consumed in about 90 min.	-MVC -Power -Cortisol and Testosterone -SHBG -CK -Leukocytes.	Squats, lower limb presses, and bilateral knee extensions were performed in 4 sets with a load of 8RM with 2 min rest.	Cross-Over	MVC was decreased after the ALC trial 12h training, MVC normalized in both groups after 24h. No differences in Jump performance; Cortisol was higher at 12 at 24h in the high dose group. Neither testosterone or SHBG were influenced by ALC. Free testosterone was lower in the high dose group at 12 and 24h. No differences in the CK for any group. No differences in leukocytes.

Table 1. *Cont.*

Author [Ref] (Year)	n	Aim	Alcohol (dose)	Mix	Administration Time	Measures	Resistance Training	Comparator	Outcomes (Compared to Comparator)
Levitt et al. [22] (2017)	13	The effect of acute ALC consumption on muscular recovery process.	1.09 g/kg	The ALC was diluted to 15% v/v in an artificially sweetened beverage.	The beverage volume was split into 10 equal portions; one portion was administered each minute over a 10min ingestion period.	-TNF-α -Il-1β -Il-6 -Il-8 -Il-10 -Soreness -Isometric, concentric and eccentric torque -CK	300 maximal single-lower limb eccentric leg extensions.	Cross-Over	No difference in soreness. No difference in strength. No difference in CK. No difference in any cytokine.
Levitt et al. [28] (2018)	10	To investigate the effect of ALC consumed after heavy eccentric resistance exercise on measures of muscle power.	1.09 g/kg	Smirnoff 40% ALC Vodka diluted to 15% v/v in an artificially sweetened beverage.	The beverage was split into 10 equal portions and one portion consumed every 3 min during the 30-min beverage ingestion period.	-Soreness -Peak power -Peak force -Jump height	4 sets of 10 repetitions at 110% of concentric 1RM; 3 min passive rest in between sets	Cross-Over	No differences were found in peak power nor peak force or jump height. No differences were found in soreness measures.
McLeay et al. [23] (2017)	8	To investigate the effects of ALC consumption on recovery of muscle force.	0.88 g/kg	37.5% ALC/volume; Smirnoff Vodka in orange juice	Six drinks were consumed every 15 min over 1.5 hr.	-CK -Soreness -Isometric, concentric and eccentric torque.	300 maximal single-lower limb eccentric leg extensions through a 60° ROM at an angular speed of 30°/s.	Cross-Over	No difference in isometric, concentric and eccentric torque. No difference in CK. No difference in muscle soreness.
Murphy et al. [24] (2013)	9	To evaluate the effects of ALC ingestion on lower-body strength and power and physiological and cognitive recovery	1g/kg	37.5% ALC/volume; Smirnoff Vodka in orange juice (ratio 3.2:1).	An equal volume of beverage was consumed every 20 min over a total time of 150 min	-RPE -CMJ -MVC -Urine -CK -CRP -Cortisol and Testosterone -Cognitive function	Rugby match	Cross-Over	No difference in RPE. No differences in CMJ and MVC. No difference in CK and CRP. No difference in testosterone. Large effect size for cortisol increase after 16h in the ALC group. Larger urine volume after night in the ALC group. Decreased cognitive function was observed in the ALC group.

43

Table 1. *Cont.*

Author [Ref] (Year)	n	Aim	Alcohol (dose)	Mix	Administration Time	Measures	Resistance Training	Comparator	Outcomes (Compared to Comparator)
Parr et al. [9] (2014)	8	Evaluate the effect of ALC intake on rates of myofibrillar protein synthesis following strenuous exercise	-1.5g/kg with CHO -1.5g/kg with PRO	Vodka and Orange juice (ratio 1:4)	6 equal volumes were consumed during a 3 h period.	-Biopsy -Blood glucose -Plasma AA concentration -Intracellular signalling proteins	8×5 at 80% of 1RM -10×30 s high intensity intervals at 110% of PPO; 3 min rest between sets	Cross-Over	Blood ALC was higher in the PRO group after 6 and 8h after consumption. Blood Glucose was higher in the ALC-CHO group after 5h.AA (EEA and BCAA) were lower in the ALC groups compared to the no ALC group.mTOR phosphorylation was higher in the no ALC group at 2 and 8h post exercise. p70S6kphosphorylation was higher in the no ALC and the ALC-PRO group at 8h post exercise. Muscle protein synthesis was greater in the No ALC group than the ALC-PRO, which was greater than the ALC-CHO group.
Poulsen et al. [25] (2007)	19	Evaluate acute ALC intoxication on skeletal muscle function	1.5 g/L	ALC 96% with orange juice (ratio 1:4)	5 doses with intervals of 1h each.	-CK -Ca^{2+} -Strength -Endurance	MVC Isokinetic endurance and isometric knee extensors (30 extensions at a velocity of 180°/s)	Cross-Over	No differences in strength and endurance. No differences in CK. Small reduction in Ca^{2+} only in the ALC group.
Vingren et al. [26] (2013)	8	To examine the testosterone bioavailability and the anabolic endocrine milieu in response to acute ethanol ingestion	1.09 g/kg	ALC was diluted to a concentration of 19% v/v absolute ethanol in an artificially sweetened and calorie-free beverage	The participants drank 1/10 of the drink each minute during a 10-min ingestion period.	-HR -RPE -Testosterone -SHBG -Lactate -Cortisol -Estradiol	6×10 squats starting at 80% of 1 RM and 2 min of rest between sets.	Cross-Over	No difference in HR, RPE and lactate. Serum testosterone and free testosterone was higher for ALC at 300min post exercise. FAI was higher in the ALC group. No difference in cortisol levels. No differences in estradiol.
Tot.	127		Mean 1.1g/kg						

N= Number of participants; g/L= grams per liter; g/kg= grams per kilogram; ALC= Alcohol; CK= Creatine kinase; Ca^{2+} = Calcium; MVC= Maximum voluntary contraction; ROM= Range of movement; HR= Heart rate; RPE= Rating of perceived exertion; CMJ= Counter movement jump; HPO= Horizontal power output; RE= Resistance exercise; SHBG= Sex hormone-binding globulin; RM= Repetition maximum; CRP= C-reactive protein; CHO= carbohydrate; PRO= Protein; AA= Amino Acids; PPO= Peak power output; EAA = Essential amino acids; BCAA= Branched Chain amino acids; FAI= Free androgen index.

3.1.5. Urine Measures

Only Murphy et al. [24] included urine measures. Post-intervention urine output, nude mass and urine-specific gravity were measured. No differences were found for nude mass and urine-specific gravity between conditions. The ALC group had an increased total volume output overnight when compared to the NO-ALC group.

3.1.6. Cortisol

Four studies included measures of cortisol [19,21,24,26]. In the study of Barnes et al. [19] the cortisol levels increased after 12h after treatment in both conditions, after which at 24h returned to baseline levels. A second rise in cortisol was seen at 36h under the ALC condition but not in the NO-ALC condition. Haugvard et al. [21] showed that no differences were shown between the two conditions at any specific time point after the intervention (12 and 24 h post-treatment). However, if the 12 and 24 h cortisol values were combined and averaged, these resulted to be significantly elevated only in the ALC condition at 24 h after the intervention. Murphy et al. [24] showed that a significant decrease post-match was followed by a significant increase at 16h post intervention. No difference was found in the levels of cortisol between the two interventions. However, a large effect size was found between the %change from 2 to 16 h post-match for the increase in cortisol response after ALC consumption. Vingren et al. [26] found that cortisol levels were not affected by ALC post intervention. Cortisol was elevated immediately after, after 20, 40, 60, 120, 140 and 300 min post-intervention in both ALC and NO-ALC conditions.

3.1.7. Testosterone

Four studies included measures of cortisol [19,21,24,26]. In the study of Barnes et al. [19] no difference in the testosterone levels compared to baseline ware seen at any time point after the intervention in either two conditions (12-24-36 and 48 h after the intervention). In the study of Haugvard et al. [21] the levels of testosterone were not altered across trials neither for the ALC and the NO-ALC condition. Calculated free testosterone (testosterone/SHBG multiplied by a factor of 10) was not different between trials. However, if the measures at 12 and 24 h after the intervention were combined and averaged the levels of testosterone resulted to be lower only in the ALC condition after 24 h. Murphy et al. [24] showed that a reduction in testosterone was present after 2 h post-match followed by a significant increase 16h post-match. However, no differences were shown between the testosterone levels for the two conditions neither between %changes from 2 to 16 h post-match. Vingren et al. [26] found a significant effect for treatment for testosterone in which the levels were increased immediately and 140 and 300 min after the intervention for the ALC group, whereas it appeared to be decreased in the NO-ALC group between 60 and 300 min post-intervention. Free testosterone also seemed to be increased between 60 and 300 min post-intervention for both conditions.

3.1.8. Estradiol

Only one study included measures of estradiol after ALC consumption [26]. The study indicates that the levels of estradiol were elevated immediately after and between 20 and 40 min after the intervention, when compared to baseline measures, in both groups, with no significant differences between the ALC and the NO-ALC group. The results underlie that ALC has no effect on estradiol during recovery from RT.

3.1.9. Sexual Hormone Binding Globulin

Two studies included measures of SHBG [21,26]. In none of the included records the levels of SHBG seemed to be altered by ALC intake, neither by the acute bouts of exercise proposed by the two authors. ALC does not seem to be a modulating factor for SHBG following RE.

3.1.10. Leukocytes and Cytokines

Three of the included studies included measures of leukocytes and cytokines [19,21,22]. Barnes performed analysis of total and differential leukocytes and found that total, neutrophil and monocyte concentration increased after the intervention but decreased to baseline values after 12h. However, no difference was present between the two conditions. Haugvard et al. [21] found no difference between conditions regarding the white blood cell, neutrophils or monocytes count. Following RE both conditions showed a sub-clinical leucocytosis 1h post-exercise. Levitt et al. [22] analysed inflammatory markers in women post-exercise, in particular TNF-α, IL-1β, IL-6, IL-8 and IL-10 before, at 5, 24 and 48h post-intervention.IL-10, IL-8 and TNF-α increased after the intervention in both groups. IL-6 and IL-1β remained unchanged over time for both conditions. No differences for cytokine was present between the ALC and the NO-ALC condition. ALC doesn't seem to affect neither leukocytes nor cytokines after RE during recovery.

3.1.11. C-reactive Protein

C-reactive protein was evaluated only in the study of Murphy et al. [24], in which however no significant difference was highlighted neither regarding time, when data was compared to baseline, neither regarding condition, when ALC and NO-ALC where compared. The findings indicate that post-match alcohol consumption did not unduly affect CRP markers of damage.

3.1.12. Plasma Amino Acids

Plasma amino acids (AA) have been included only in the study of Parr et al. [9], who evaluated EEA, BCAA and leucine at 0, 1, 2, 4, 6 and 8 h after alcohol consumption following RE. It has to be noted that Parr administered a concentration of alcohol in conjunction with either CHO or PRO. The results were then compared to a control group who did not ingest ALC but consumed a single dose of 25 g of whey protein.

A significant effect for time and treatment were found. At all-time points the NO-ALC group had significantly higher levels of essential AA (EEA), branched chain AA (BCAA) and leucine compared to the ALC-PRO group. Both groups (the NO-ALC and the ALC-PRO) had at all-time points significantly higher levels of AA compared to the ALC-CHO group. No difference in the levels of AA compared to baseline was shown, at any time point, in the ALC-CHO group. Leucine, EEA and BCAA were elevated compared to baseline at 1 and 6 h post-ALC ingestion for the NO-ALC and ALC-PRO group. The data from the study of Parr et al. [9] indicates that ALC alone does not influence the levels of plasma AA, however can be a factor that limits the rise of blood concentration of AA following protein consumption.

3.1.13. Intracellular Signaling Proteins and Rates of Muscle Protein Synthesis

mTOR, p70S6K, eEF2, 4E-BP1, AMPK, MuRF-1 mRNA and fractional synthetic rate of myofibrillar protein synthesis were analysed in the study of Parr et al. [9]. ALC and NO-ALC consumption modalities have been described in the previous subsection. mTOR^{Ser2448} phosphorylation was higher in all groups at 2h post treatment. However, mTOR phosphorylation in the NO-ALC group was higher than the ALC-CHO (76%) and ALC-PRO (54%) group at 2 and 8 h post-exercise. p70S6K phosphorylation was greater after 2h post-exercise compared to baseline only in the NO-ALC and the ALC-PRO groups. No differences were shown for the ALC-CHO group. eEF2 phosphorylation decreased below rest values at 2 and 8 h in the ALC-CHO and ALC-PRO groups. No differences were shown for the NO-ALC group at any time point.

No differences for time and condition were shown for 4E-BP1$^{Thr37/46}$ or AMPK^{Thr172} phosphorylation. There were increases above rest in MuRF-1 mRNA at 2 h post- intervention with no differences between treatments. All values returned to baseline at 8h post- intervention.

Fractional synthetic rate of myofibrillar protein synthesis were increased above baseline for all groups from 2 to 8 h post-intervention. However, a hierarchical reduction was shown when data was compared to the NO-ALC group in the ALC-PRO (-24% compared to NO-ALC) and ALC-CHO (−38% compared NO-ALC and −18% compared to ALC-PRO) groups. Data suggests that ALC consumption impairs the response of muscle protein synthesis during recovery despite optimal nutrient provision.

3.1.14. Calcium

Only one study has evaluated the effects of ALC on Ca^{2+} via blood sampling [25]. The authors report that the Ca^{2+} levels were similar before exercise for both conditions. A decrease of approximately 2% was observed following the exercise bouts. A further decrease was observed in the ALC condition, and the difference with the NO-ALC condition was significant only after the strength evaluation. Hypocalcaemia was not induced by ALC and no differences were shown for resting free Ca^{2+} levels indicating that free Ca^{2+} concentrations were not affected by alcohol per se.

3.2. Physical Measures

3.2.1. Force

Nine studies have examined the effects of post-exercise ALC consumption on force [18,20–25,27,28]. McLeay et al. [23] evaluated maximal isometric, concentric and eccentric muscular contractions of the quadriceps femoris using an isokinetic dynamometer for both lower limbs using one lower limb as control. A significant difference between lower limbs was present post-treatment (exercised vs. non-exercised lower limb) up to 60 h post-exercise regarding maximal isometric tension, concentric and eccentric torque but no difference was observed between the ALC and the NO-ALC condition. Barnes et al. [18,27] in both studies evaluated isometric, concentric and eccentric contractions of the quadriceps muscles of both lower limbs using one lower limb as control. Isometric tension was measured at 75° of knee angle. Concentric and eccentric torque was measured at an angular speed of 30°/s. In both studies a decrease in performance was seen in both the ALC and NO-ALC groups over time in the exercised lower limb for all the evaluated measures (isometric and eccentric peak torques as well as for isometric, concentric and eccentric average peak torques). A greater decrease in performance was however seen in the ALC group in the first study [27] at 36h post-intervention (isometric and eccentric peak torques were reduced 39 and 44% compared to pre-exercise measures, respectively, with ALC whereas losses of 29 and 27% for the same measures in the NO-ALC group. Average peak torque was reduced by 41% (isometric), 43% (concentric) and 45% (eccentric) with ALC compared to 29, 32 and 26% with NO-ALC groups, respectively), while no differences were seen between 36 and 60h post-intervention. In the second study [18], except for average peak isometric torque, all measures were different between interventions with the greatest decrements observed in the ALC group. Greatest decreases in peak torque were observed at 36 h with losses of 12%, 28% and 19% occurring in the NO-ALC group for isometric, concentric and eccentric contractions, respectively. Peak torque loss was significantly larger in ALC with the same performance measures decreasing by 34%, 40% and 34%). Levitt et al. [22] measured peak torque for the knee extension exercise on each lower limb using an isokinetic dynamometer. The same assessment procedure used by Barnes et al. [18,27] was adopted. A reduction post-intervention was found for peak isometric, concentric and eccentric torque between the exercised and not-exercised lower limb, but no difference was found between the ALC and NO-ALC condition immediately post nor at 24 and 48 h post-intervention. Poulsen et al. [25] evaluated isokinetic muscle strength of the dominant knee extensors and non-dominant wrist flexors. No differences in isometric strength was observed immediately post, 4, 24 or 48 h post intervention, neither regarding time, when compared to baseline, neither regarding ALC condition. Murphy et al. [24] measured peak MVC of the knee extensors and found that a significant reduction compared to baseline was evident at all measured time points (2 and 16 h post-intervention), but no differences were present between the ALC and NO-ALC group. Haugvad et al. [21] have also measured isometric

MVC of the knee extensors and the results reported by the authors showed stable values in all analysed conditions (Low ALC dose, High ALC dose and NO-ALC). A decrease immediately after performance and a recovery from immediately after to 12 and 24 h post intervention was seen in all groups, with no significant differences between trials. Clarkson et al. [20] measured isometric strength of the elbow flexors and the results are similar to those of Haugvad et al. with a reduction immediately post-exercise but no difference between conditions. The level of isometric strength returned to baseline 5 days post-intervention. Except for the studies of Barnes et al. no differences seem to be present following ALC consumption on force during recovery following RE. It has to be noted that the ALC dose provided by Barnes et al. is of 1g/kg, which is neither the minimum or maximum dose provided across the studies.

3.2.2. Power

Four studies [19,24,28,30] included measures of power following ALC consumption and RE. Barnes et al. [19] have included measures of counter movement jump (CMJ) and horizontal power output (HPO). HPO did not vary neither over time neither regarding condition. CMJ instead showed a significant time x treatment effect, where a decrease in jump performance was observed after 24 and 48 h post-intervention only in the ALC group. However, the authors underline that the decrements seen in performance are trivial as the decrease in the jumping performance of the CMJ was a mean value of 12 cm. Murphy et al. [24] have included a measure of CMJ over time, where each participant was required to perform 10-maximal repeated CMJs. The results of Murphy et al. do not show any difference neither regarding time neither regarding condition. Levitt et al. [28] have included measures of vertical power, and similarly to Barnes et al., the reported measures of power show a time effect, with a reduction in vertical power output after 24 and 48 h post-intervention, but no effect regarding condition. Haugvad et al. [21] included a measure of squat jump performed without any counter movement on a force platform. Jump height was calculated for analysis. Jump height was reduced immediately after and 12 h post-intervention in all groups (low-ALC, high-ALC and NO-ALC condition). However, no difference between any group was present. ALC doesn't seem to have an effect on power output, at least in the 48 h following its consumption.

3.2.3. Muscular Endurance

Maximal isokinetic muscular endurance was calculated for the dominant knee extensors and non-dominant wrist in the study of Poulsen et al. [25] using an isokinetic dynamometer. Thirty maximal reciprocal movements were performed at a velocity of 180°/s without any rest interval. Subjects were instructed to exert maximal effort in every single movement and not to economise the muscle exertion. An endurance index was calculated defined as the mean-peak torque of the last five repetitions as a percentage of the mean-peak torque of the first five repetitions. The results obtained by the authors show no differences in muscular endurance 4, 24 and 48h after treatment neither after ALC intoxication neither in the NO-ALC group. No changes were evident neither in the leg extensors neither in the wrist flexors or between the endurance index for both conditions for both muscle groups. The results were also stratified according to gender and similar findings were achieved.

3.2.4. Soreness

Five studies included measures of soreness [18,20,22,23,28]. Barnes et al. [18] evaluated soreness by asking each participant at different time points their levels of soreness by giving a value from 0 (no pain) to 10 (worst possible pain). Soreness was rated while stepping up (concentric muscular contraction) onto a 40 cm box and lowering into a squatting position. Clarkson et al. [20] evaluated soreness by questionnaire, measured for the forearm flexor muscles, using a scale of 1 to 10. Levitt et al. [22] measured soreness applying on the vastuslateralis, in three different points along the muscle belly, a pressure of 35N. Each participant rated the pain giving a value from 0 to 10. In a subsequent study Levitt et al. [28] evaluated pain by asking the participants to self-report their level of pain using a scale from 0 to 5. McLeay et al. [23] used the same protocol as above described in the study of Barnes et al. [18]. All the retrieved records show a time effect for muscle soreness related to the intervention protocol, with increases over a period of 24 and 48 h after the training intervention, with no differences between the ALC and the NO-ALC condition. The results indicate that RT is a factor responsible to increase muscle soreness between 24 and 48 h post training, whereas ALC consumption is not.

3.2.5. Rate of Perceived Exertion

Rates of perceived exertion were measured in three of the retrieved studies [19,24,26]. The study of Vingren [26], was the only one evaluating RPE before and after a single session of static RE. Barnes and Murphy [19,24] evaluated RPE before and after a rugby match. In particular Murphy et al. evaluated RPE after a competitive rugby league game, whereas Barnes et al. after a simulated rugby match. The results of Vingren and Murphy highlight a significant time effect, with increases of RPE after the RT and the rugby league game, but no significant differences between the RPE of the ALC or the NO-ALC groups. The results of Barnes et al. are in line to those of the previous authors regarding the time effect of RPE following the exercising protocol, however a difference was shown between conditions. The ALC group reported lower levels of RPE at the end of the third quarter of the simulated game, compared to the NO-ALC group at the same time measurement. Despite the significant results, the mean difference between the two conditions is very small (ALC=15.2 ± 1.6; NO-ALC=16.5 ± 1.2) and not present at any other time point.

3.3. Cognitive Function

Cognitive function was assessed only in the study of Murphy et al. [24] through a modified version of the Stroop test. This test of cognitive function was a computer-based program requiring subjects to react to repeated color and word stimuli. The program analyzed response time and accuracy for congruent and incongruent stimuli. Measures of cognitive function were recorded before, immediately post, 2 and 16 h intervention. The results provided by the authors show no difference over time for cognition test time, congruent reaction time, or incongruent reaction time. However, the time required to complete the cognition test significantly increased in the ALC compared to the NO-ALC group and a large ES was shown for increased cognition test time, congruent and incongruent reaction time in the ALC group compared to the NO-ALC group. The findings indicate that ALC consumption impairs cognitive function during recovery, which may be a negative factor in sports where decision making processes, speed and quality of responses to visual stimuli (especially team sports) are essential.

4. Discussion

By evaluating the effects of alcohol consumption on recovery following RE from biological, physical and cognitive perspective, we have been able to provide a comprehensive description of the multifactorial nature of alcohol consumption. Indeed, alcohol consumption is a common occurrence in the general population on global scale and it is a phenomenon that has not been explored in depth when it comes to post-exercise recovery, even more so in RE post-exercise recovery. The main findings highlight that ALC cannot be considered as a modulating factor for the majority of the retrieved biological measures. In fact, creatine kinase, heart rate, lactate, blood glucose, estradiol, sexual hormone binding globulin, leukocytes and cytokines, C-reactive protein and calcium do not seem to be modified following ALC consumption during the acute recovery phase post-resistance exercise. Only cortisol levels seem to be increased, conversely testosterone, plasma amino acids, and rates of muscle protein synthesis decreased. When considering the retrieved physical measures force, power, muscular endurance, soreness and rate of perceived exertion also seem to be unmodified following alcohol consumption during recovery. The general findings therefore highlight that muscle function is not altered by alcohol consumption following exercise bouts, however the altered endocrinological asset regarding cortisol and testosterone and the consequent suppressed rates of muscular protein synthesis and reduced circulating levels of amino acids, suggest that long-term muscular adaptations could be impaired.

A trend of heart rate increase following the exercise intervention has been detected, however no difference was shown between the ALC and the NO-ALC condition. This conclusion raises different concerns since alcohol acts as a diuretic and it contributes to faster elimination of water content from the bloodstream, leading to increased viscous blood plasma which is harder to pump and deliver to the body tissues [31]. The heart has to adapt to these conditions to increase the cardiac output. There seems to be a dose response relationship between the alcohol consumption and heart rate i.e., there is a positive correlation between alcohol consumption and heart rate response [32]. Consequently, this has the potential to alter individual RPE [33]. This latter parameter also seems to not be influenced by alcohol consumption. Only one of the retrieved studies has shown there was a difference between the ALC and NO-ALC group with the ALC group showing less perceived exertion compared to the NO-ALC group.

As previously stated alcohol acts as a diuretic and thus can explain why in the study of Murphy at al [24] the ALC group had an increased total volume output overnight when compared to the NO-ALC group.

One of the most interesting findings of this review was found in the study by Parr et al. [9] who demonstrated that blood glucose is affected by CHO but not ALC during recovery after RE. This is in alignment with findings of Lustig [34] who claims that toxic effects of alcohol are very similar to excessive sugar exposure mainly for its fructose content. Even though fructose does not show the same acute toxic effects of ethanol, it encompasses all the chronic hazardous effects on long-term health [34].

Creatine kinase was also unmodified by ALC consumption. Such enzyme which is present in the muscles, when detectable in the peripheral circulation, is commonly used as a measure of muscle damage [8]. None of the authors which reported measures of CK showed differences between groups, instead correlations were established between the ALC and the NO-ALC condition. ALC cannot be considered as a modulating factor for CK following RE and the increases of CK shown are the result of muscle damage following the exercise bouts. Neither leukocytes nor cytokines seem to be changed following alcohol consumption, which means that the inflammatory response is not modulated by alcohol consumption. Such is a controversial finding because as reported by different authors [35,36] alcohol abuse not only increases inflammation but also alters the immune function of the body. Probably healthy individuals, who regularly exercise, as those included in each study of this review, do not express altered inflammatory or immune function following a single acute alcohol intoxication. Same trend is shown by CRP, which confirms that muscle damage and inflammation are not dependent, in the analyzed population, from the ingestion of alcohol [24]. Such findings may also explain why perceived soreness was not different between the ALC and NO-ALC groups analyzed.

Cortisol and testosterone levels during post RE when compared between ALC and NO-ALC groups appear to be altered. On average, the participants who consumed ALC expressed higher levels of cortisol and lower levels of testosterone in comparison to the NO-ALC group. Decreased levels of testosterone and increased levels of cortisol are suggested to be indicative for a disturbance in the anabolic-catabolic balance, which likely leads to decreased recovery and therefore, decreased levels of performance [24,37]. When present in excessive levels, cortisol is an overall catabolic hormone, which decreases lean body and muscle mass and increases energy expenditure [38]. Conversely, testosterone is an anabolic hormone, which may also explain why in the study of Parr et al. mTOR phosphorylation in the NO-ALC group was higher than the ALC-CHO (76%) and ALC-PRO (54%) group at 2 and 8 h post-exercise. In addition, also rates of muscle protein synthesis were higher in the NO-ALC group when compared to those who ingested ALC. However, muscle protein synthesis may also appear decreased because of the decreased plasma levels of AA showed following ALC consumption. These findings can have major implications with regards to the recovery and performance of both non athletes and professional athletes. An acute bout of vigorous RE can result in a transient increase in protein turnover and until feeding, protein balance remains negative [39,40]. Protein ingestion post exercise enhances muscle protein synthesis and net protein balance [41] by increasing myofibrillar protein fraction with RE [42], but as seen in the study of Parr et al. alcohol ingestion after RE has the ability to disrupt this process. Beyond physical aspects, decreased protein synthesis leads to impaired long-term memory in humans [43–45], which can be particularly important in professional athletes who have many cognitive demands with respect to both short and long term memory [17].

In regards to measures of force only study of Barnes et al. [18] showed that following ALC consumption the levels of isometric, concentric and eccentric torque decreased, while other studies in this review that measured force production showed no differences between the ALC and NO-ALC groups during recovery following RE. As depicted in the results section, with respect to muscle function and force, only study by Barnes et al. has shown that moderate consumption of alcohol can amplify the loss of force associated with strenuous eccentric exercise [18]. This particular study detected significant decrements in average peak isometric, concentric and eccentric torques at 36 h post-exercise [18]. Clearly more research is needed since the outcomes among the mentioned studies are quite distinct. All measures of force were assessed from 2 h to 48 h post RT or ALC ingestion and the measures all appear decreased because of the exercise performed. The retrieved measures of performance returned to baseline within 2 days following both ALC consumption and the exercise bouts. Same trend is shown for the other two measures of performance retrieved: power and muscular endurance which decreased following the exercise bouts in both groups with no difference between those who consumed ALC and those who did not.

Several limitations have been encountered during the realization of this manuscript. Firstly, a very limited body of evidence was present within each screened database, on the topic of alcohol consumption following bouts of RE, therefore it is not possible to consider such review comprehensive and definitive. Few studies have evaluated in depth biological measures of protein synthesis or specific markers of muscular function. Other important limitation is the timely evaluation of each study. Each included measure was evaluated in a timeframe ranging from 2 h to 48h post exercise or alcohol consumption. Therefore, only acute modifications were evaluated and it was not possible to consider hormonal fluctuations beyond 2 days and their relative effects. Lastly, the total sample size of each study was small ranging between 8 and 19 participants.

5. Conclusions

Alcohol consumption following resistance exercise doesn't seem to affect the majority of the retrieved biological and physical measures. However, levels of cortisol were increased, and levels testosterone and rates of muscle protein synthesis were decreased, which indicates that long term muscular adaptations could be impaired if alcohol consumption during recovery is consistent. Muscle function doesn't seem to be influenced by alcohol consumption during recovery. Studies with larger cohorts evaluating the effects of alcohol consumption during recovery following resistance exercise are needed to further understand the long-term effects of alcohol ingestion.

Supplementary Materials: Supplementary materials can be found at http://www.mdpi.com/2411-5142/4/3/41/s1.

Author Contributions: Conceptualization, N.L.; Methodology, N.L.; Writing – Original Draft Preparation, N.L.; Writing – Review & Editing, N.L;

Funding: This research received no external funding.

Acknowledgments: I would like to thank Kaltrina Feka and Valerio Giustino from PhD program in Health Promotion and Cognitive Sciences at University of Palermo for helping me to do the article search and assess risk of bias.

Conflicts of Interest: The author declares no conflict of interest.

References

1. Schoenfeld, B. *Science and Development of Muscle Hypertrophy.* 2016. Available online: http://public.eblib.com/choice/publicfullrecord.aspx?p=4746185 (accessed on 13 May 2019).
2. Kraemer, W.; Ratamess, N. Physiology of resistance training: Current issues. *Orthop. Physic. Ther. Clin. N. Am.* **2000**, *9*, 467–513.

3. Harries, S.K.; Lubans, D.R.; Callister, R. Resistance training to improve power and sports performance in adolescent athletes: A systematic review and meta-analysis. *J. Sci. Med. Sport* **2012**, *15*, 532–540. [CrossRef] [PubMed]
4. American College of Sports. American College of Sports Medicine position stand. Progression models in resistance training for healthy adults. *Med. Sci. Sports Exerc.* **2009**, *41*, 687–708. [CrossRef] [PubMed]
5. Hausswirth, C. *Recovery for Performance in Sport*; Human Kinetics: Champaign, IL, USA, 2019.
6. Barnett, A. Using recovery modalities between training sessions in elite athletes: Does it help? *Sports Med.* **2006**, *36*, 781–796. [CrossRef] [PubMed]
7. Halson, S. Recovery techniques for athletes. *Aspetar Sports Med. J.* **2013**, *26*, 1–6.
8. Vella, L.D.; Cameron-Smith, D. Alcohol, athletic performance and recovery. *Nutrients* **2010**, *2*, 781–789. [CrossRef]
9. Parr, E.B.; Camera, D.M.; Areta, J.L.; Burke, L.M.; Phillips, S.M.; Hawley, J.A.; Coffey, V.G. Alcohol ingestion impairs maximal post-exercise rates of myofibrillar protein synthesis following a single bout of concurrent training. *PLoS ONE* **2014**, *9*, e88384. [CrossRef] [PubMed]
10. Barnes, M.J. Alcohol: Impact on sports performance and recovery in male athletes. *Sports Med.* **2014**, *44*, 909–919. [CrossRef] [PubMed]
11. Mager, A. 'White liquor hits black livers': Meanings of excessive liquor consumption in South Africa in the second half of the twentieth century. *Soc. Sci. Med.* **2004**, *59*, 735–751. [CrossRef]
12. Miguez, H.A. Epidemiology of alcohol consumption in Argentina. *Vertex* **2003**, *14*, 19–26.
13. Pretorius, L.; Naidoo, A.; Reddy, S.P. "Kitchen cupboard drinking": A review of South African women's secretive alcohol addiction, treatment history, and barriers to accessing treatment. *Soc. Work Public Health* **2009**, *24*, 89–99. [CrossRef] [PubMed]
14. Rachdaoui, N.; Sarkar, D.K. Effects of alcohol on the endocrine system. *Endocrinol. Metab. Clin. N. Am.* **2013**, *42*, 593–615. [CrossRef] [PubMed]
15. Lang, C.H.; Pruznak, A.M.; Nystrom, G.J.; Vary, T.C. Alcohol-induced decrease in muscle protein synthesis associated with increased binding of mTOR and raptor: Comparable effects in young and mature rats. *Nutr. Metab.* **2009**, *6*, 4. [CrossRef] [PubMed]
16. Vary, T.C.; Frost, R.A.; Lang, C.H. Acute alcohol intoxication increases atrogin-1 and MuRF1 mRNA without increasing proteolysis in skeletal muscle. *Am. J. Physiol. Regul. Integr. Comp. Physiol.* **2008**, *294*, R1777–R1789. [CrossRef] [PubMed]
17. Downs, S.H.; Black, N. The feasibility of creating a checklist for the assessment of the methodological quality both of randomised and non-randomised studies of health care interventions. *J. Epidemiol. Commun. Health* **1998**, *52*, 377–384. [CrossRef] [PubMed]
18. Barnes, M.J.; Mundel, T.; Stannard, S.R. Acute alcohol consumption aggravates the decline in muscle performance following strenuous eccentric exercise. *J. Sci. Med. Sport* **2010**, *13*, 189–193. [CrossRef] [PubMed]
19. Barnes, M.J.; Mundel, T.; Stannard, S.R. The effects of acute alcohol consumption on recovery from a simulated rugby match. *J. Sports Sci.* **2012**, *30*, 295–304. [CrossRef] [PubMed]
20. Clarkson, P.M.; Reichsman, F. The effect of ethanol on exercise-induced muscle damage. *J. Stud. Alcohol* **1990**, *51*, 19–23. [CrossRef]
21. Haugvad, A.; Haugvad, L.; Hamarsland, H.; Paulsen, G. Ethanol Does Not Delay Muscle Recovery, but Decreases the Testosterone: Cortisol Ratio. *Med. Sci. Sports Exerc.* **2014**, *46*, 2175–2183. [CrossRef]
22. Levitt, D.E.; Hiu-Ying, L.; Duplanty, A.A.; McFarlin, B.K.; Hill, D.W.; Vingreen, J.L. Effect of alcohol after muscle-damaging resistance exercise on muscular performance recovery and inflammatory capacity in women. *Eur. J. Appl. Physiol.* **2017**, *117*, 1195–1206. [CrossRef]
23. McLeay, Y.; Stannard, S.R.; Mundel, L.; Foskett, A.; Barnes, M. Effect of Alcohol Consumption on Recovery From Eccentric Exercise Induced Muscle Damage in Females. *Int. J. Sport. Nutr. Exerc. Metab.* **2017**, *27*, 115–121. [CrossRef] [PubMed]
24. Murphy, A.P.; Snape, A.E.; Minett, G.M.; Skein, M.; Duffield, R. The effect of post-match alcohol ingestion on recovery from competitive rugby league matches. *J. Strength Cond. Res.* **2013**, *27*, 1304–1312. [CrossRef] [PubMed]
25. Poulsen, M.B.; Jakobsen, J.; Aagaard, N.K.; Andersen, H. Motor performance during and following acute alcohol intoxication in healthy non-alcoholic subjects. *Eur. J. Appl. Physiol.* **2007**, *101*, 513–523. [CrossRef] [PubMed]

26. Vingren, J.L.; Hill, D.W.; Buddhadev, H.; Duplanty, A. Postresistance exercise ethanol ingestion and acute testosterone bioavailability. *Med. Sci. Sports Exerc* **2013**, *45*, 1825–1832. [CrossRef] [PubMed]
27. Barnes, M.J.; Mundel, T.; Stannard, S.R. Post-exercise alcohol ingestion exacerbates eccentric-exercise induced losses in performance. *Eur. J. Appl. Physiol.* **2010**, *108*, 1009–1014. [CrossRef] [PubMed]
28. Levitt, D.E.; Idemudia, N.O.; Cregar, C.M.; Duplanty, A.A.; Hill, D.W.; Vingren, J.L. Alcohol after Resistance Exercise Does not Affect Muscle Power Recovery. *J. Strength Cond. Res.* **2018**. [CrossRef]
29. Kalinowski, A.; Humphreys, K. Governmental standard drink definitions and low-risk alcohol consumption guidelines in 37 countries. *Addiction* **2016**, *111*, 1293–1298. [CrossRef] [PubMed]
30. Jones, A.W. Excretion of alcohol in urine and diuresis in healthy men in relation to their age, the dose administered and the time after drinking. *Forensic Sci. Int.* **1990**, *45*, 217–224. [CrossRef]
31. Brunner, S.; Herber, R.; Drobesch, C.; Peters, A.; Massberg, S.; Kaab, S.; Sinner, M.F. Alcohol consumption, sinus tachycardia, and cardiac arrhythmias at the Munich Octoberfest: Results from the Munich Beer Related Electrocardiogram Workup Study (MunichBREW). *Eur. Heart J.* **2017**, *38*, 2100–2106. [CrossRef]
32. Borg, G.; Domserius, M.; Kaijser, L. Effect of alcohol on perceived exertion in relation to heart rate and blood lactate. *Eur. J. Appl. Physiol. Occup. Physiol.* **1990**, *60*, 382–384. [CrossRef] [PubMed]
33. Lustig, R.H. Fructose: It's "alcohol without the buzz". *Adv. Nutr.* **2013**, *4*, 226–235. [CrossRef] [PubMed]
34. Kelley, K.W.; Dantzer, R. Alcoholism and inflammation: Neuroimmunology of behavioral and mood disorders. *Brain Behav. Immun.* **2011**, *25*, S13–S20. [CrossRef] [PubMed]
35. Wang, H.J.; Zakhari, S.; Jung, M.K. Alcohol, inflammation, and gut-liver-brain interactions in tissue damage and disease development. *World J. Gastroenterol.* **2010**, *16*, 1304–1313. [CrossRef] [PubMed]
36. Hoogeveen, A.R.; Zonderland, M.L. Relationships between testosterone, cortisol and performance in professional cyclists. *Int. J. Sports Med.* **1996**, *17*, 423–428. [CrossRef] [PubMed]
37. Tataranni, P.A.; Larson, D.E.; Snitker, S.; Young, J.B.; Flatt, J.P.; Ravussin, E. Effects of glucocorticoids on energy metabolism and food intake in humans. *Am. J. Physiol.* **1996**, *271*, E317–E325. [CrossRef] [PubMed]
38. Phillips, S.M.; Van Loon, L.J. Dietary protein for athletes: From requirements to optimum adaptation. *J. Sports Sci.* **2011**, *29*, S29–S38. [CrossRef] [PubMed]
39. Rasmussen, B.B.; Tipton, K.D.; Miller, S.L.; Wolf, S.E.; Wolfe, R.R. An oral essential amino acid-carbohydrate supplement enhances muscle protein anabolism after resistance exercise. *J. Appl. Physiol.* **2000**, *88*, 386–392. [CrossRef]
40. Kraemer, W.J.; Volek, J.S.; Bush, J.A.; Putukian, M.; Sebastianelli, W.J. Hormonal responses to consecutive days of heavy-resistance exercise with or without nutritional supplementation. *J. Appl. Physiol.* **1998**, *85*, 1544–1555. [CrossRef]
41. Wilkinson, S.B.; Phillips, S.M.; Atherton, P.J.; Patel, R.; Yarasheski, K.E.; Tarnopolsky, M.A.; Rennie, M.J. Differential effects of resistance and endurance exercise in the fed state on signalling molecule phosphorylation and protein synthesis in human muscle. *J. Physiol.* **2008**, *586*, 3701–3717. [CrossRef]
42. Gibbs, M.E.; Ng, K.T. Psychobiology of memory: Towards a model of memory formation. *Biobehav. Rev.* **1977**, *1*, 113–136. [CrossRef]
43. Davis, H.P.; Spanis, C.W.; Squire, L.R. Inhibition of cerebral protein synthesis: Performance at different times after passive avoidance training. *Pharmacol. Biochem. Behav.* **1976**, *4*, 13–16. [CrossRef]
44. Hernandez, P.J.; Abel, T. The role of protein synthesis in memory consolidation: Progress amid decades of debate. *Neurobiol. Learn. Mem.* **2008**, *89*, 293–311. [CrossRef] [PubMed]
45. Faubert, J. Professional athletes have extraordinary skills for rapidly learning complex and neutral dynamic visual scenes. *Sci. Rep.* **2013**, *3*, 1154. [CrossRef] [PubMed]

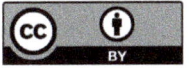

© 2019 by the author. Licensee MDPI, Basel, Switzerland. This article is an open access article distributed under the terms and conditions of the Creative Commons Attribution (CC BY) license (http://creativecommons.org/licenses/by/4.0/).

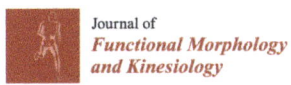

Article

Acute Cardiometabolic Responses to Multi-Modal Integrative Neuromuscular Training in Children

Avery D. Faigenbaum *, Jie Kang, Nicholas A. Ratamess, Anne C. Farrell, Mina Belfert, Sean Duffy, Cara Jenson and Jill Bush

Department of Health and Exercise Science, The College of New Jersey, Ewing, NJ 08628, USA; kang@tcnj.edu (J.K.); ratamess@tcnj.edu (N.A.R.); afarrell@tcnj.edu (A.C.F.); belferm1@tcnj.edu (M.B.); duffys1@tcnj.edu (S.D.); jensonc1@tcnj.edu (C.J.); wallacej@tcnj.edu (J.B.)
* Correspondence: faigenba@tcnj.edu; Tel.: +1-609-771-2151

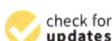

Received: 10 May 2019; Accepted: 21 June 2019; Published: 24 June 2019

Abstract: Integrative neuromuscular training (INT) has emerged as an effective strategy for improving health- and skill-related components of physical fitness, yet few studies have explored the cardiometabolic demands of this type of training in children. The aim of this study was to examine the acute cardiometabolic responses to a multi-modal INT protocol and to compare these responses to a bout of moderate-intensity treadmill (TM) walking in children. Participants ($n = 14$, age 10.7 ± 1.1 years) were tested for peak oxygen uptake (VO$_2$) and peak heart rate (HR) on a maximal TM test and subsequently participated in two experimental conditions on nonconsecutive days: a 12-min INT protocol of six different exercises performed twice for 30 s with a 30 s rest interval between sets and exercises and a 12-min TM protocol of walking at 50% VO$_2$peak. Throughout the INT protocol mean VO$_2$ and HR increased significantly from 14.9 ± 3.6 mL·kg^{-1}·min^{-1} (28.2% VO$_2$ peak) to 34.0 ± 6.4 mL·kg^{-1}·min^{-1} (64.3% VO$_2$ peak) and from 121.1 ± 9.0 bpm (61.0% HR peak) to 183.5 ± 7.9 bpm (92.4% HR peak), respectively. While mean VO$_2$ for the entire protocol did not differ between INT and TM, mean VO$_2$ and HR during selected INT exercises and mean HR for the entire INT protocol were significantly higher than TM (all $Ps \leq 0.05$). These findings suggest that INT can pose a moderate to vigorous cardiometabolic stimulus in children and selected INT exercises can be equal to or more metabolically challenging than TM walking.

Keywords: Heart rate; interval training; metabolism; oxygen consumption; physical activity; resistance training; strength training; youth

1. Introduction

A growing number of children and adolescents fail to accumulate at least 60 min of moderate to vigorous physical activity (MVPA) daily [1]. The far-reaching consequences of physical inactivity during childhood and adolescence are a constellation of cardiometabolic, musculoskeletal, and psychosocial risk factors and diseases that are challenging to manage, difficult to treat and costly to individuals and society [2]. Current efforts to increase MVPA in youth with targeted interventions have had only a small effect [3]. Notably, the impact of walking interventions on physical activity behaviors and health-related fitness measures in school-age youth have been limited [4–6]. While walking is a natural form of physical activity that is practical and inexpensive, other types of exercise may be needed to enhance cardiometabolic health, target neuromuscular deficiencies, and increase participation in MVPA. The importance of integrating different types of resistance exercise into youth fitness programs has become particularly important in light of secular declines in measures of muscular strength and power in modern day youth [7,8]. The available evidence supports a link between muscular fitness and physical activity, particularly vigorous intensity physical activity, in children and adolescents [9].

Integrative neuromuscular training (INT) is a type of exercise characterized by intermittent bouts of different strength- and skill-building exercises that are designed to improve fundamental movement skills, increase muscular fitness and prepare participants for exercise and sport activities [10]. INT has emerged as an effective strategy for improving health- and skill-related components of physical fitness in school-age youth, [11–13], and limited evidence suggests that this type of training may also offer cardiometabolic benefits [14,15]. Previous studies investigating the effects of INT on children have found significant improvements in sprinting, running, jumping, throwing and lifting performance following 8 to 10 weeks of training [11,12,16]. However, it is also important to examine the acute cardiometabolic responses to INT because the amount of time youth spend in vigorous physical activity is more strongly associated with positive health outcomes than light or moderate-intensity physical activity [17–19]. An analysis of accelerometer data from a large sample of children found vigorous physical activity was strongly associated with metabolic health whereas associations of light to moderate physical activity were weak to moderate [18]. While research evidence supports the safety, efficacy and feasibility of INT for children [11,12,16], the acute cardiometabolic responses to INT are poorly understood.

Researchers examined the acute cardiometabolic responses to a single-mode interval training protocol with medicine balls [14] or battling ropes [15] in children and found that this type of exercise can pose a potent cardiometabolic stimulus. For example, mean heart rate (HR) and oxygen uptake (VO_2) values during a 10-min bout of medicine ball interval training ranged from 61.1% to 89.6% of HR peak and from 28.2% to 63.5% of VO_2 peak [14]. Similarly, others found that the acute responses to a 12-min session of resistance training or intermittent noncontact boxing in early adolescents could be characterized as "vigorous" and therefore contribute to daily moderate to vigorous physical activity (MVPA) recommendations [20]. Due to the increasing interest in high-intensity interval training and the potential for multi-modal INT to modulate disease risk factors and improve health outcomes in youth [10,21,22], there is strong rational to further examine the acute cardiometabolic responses to INT in youth. Of relevance to the current study, strategic efforts to strengthen and improve physical education and physical activity opportunities with novel and time efficient exercise interventions are needed to increase MVPA in school-age youth and foster a healthy generation [23].

To the authors' knowledge, no previous study has examined the acute cardiometabolic responses to multi-modal INT in children and direct comparisons between INT and traditional exercise interventions such as walking have not been reported. While brisk walking can offer health benefits for children, INT has been found to enhance cardiometabolic health and neuromuscular fitness in youth [11–13]. Additional research on the acute responses to INT could be used to establish preliminary cardiometabolic references values for INT and inform the design of novel exercise interventions for children. Therefore, the purpose of this study was to examine the acute cardiometabolic responses to a multi-modal INT protocol in children and to compare these responses to a bout of moderate-intensity treadmill walking. Based on previous findings regarding the acute cardiometabolic responses to different exercise modalities in youth [14,15], we hypothesized that selected INT exercises would elicit a cardiometabolic response that was equal to or greater than brisk walking in children.

2. Materials and Methods

2.1. Participants

A convenience sample of 14 healthy children (8 boys and 6 girls; mean ± SD age 10.7 ± 1.1 years; height 143.2 ± 6.8 cm and body mass 36.3 ± 9.9 kg) volunteered to participate in this study. Participants were active members of local sports teams (primarily soccer and lacrosse), but none participated regularly in resistance training. Parents completed a modified physical activity readiness questionnaire to evaluate the health status of the participants and assess the safety for performing vigorous exercise. All parents signed a parental permission form and all participants signed a child assent form and were

2.2. Peak Aerobic Capacity Testing

All participants reported to the Human Performance Laboratory at least 2 h postprandial for peak aerobic capacity testing. VO$_2$ peak was assessed using the Fitkids treadmill test protocol [24] and a metabolic system (MedGraphics ULTIMA Metabolic System, MedGraphics Corporation, St. Paul, MN, USA). The Fitkids treadmill test is a valid and reproducible exercise test for children that consists of 90 s stages with incremental increases in speed and incline until volitional exhaustion [24]. Breath-by-breath VO$_2$ data were obtained and VO$_2$ peak was determined by recording the highest measure observed during the test [25]. HR was monitored using a soft chest strap with a HR sensor (Model A300; Polar Electro Inc., Woodbury, NY, USA). HR peak was defined as the highest value achieved during the test. Participants were asked to manually signal without verbalizing their rating of perceived exertion (RPE) during the test [26]. Prior to testing, height was measured to the nearest 0.1 cm using a wall-mounted stadiometer and body mass was measured to the nearest 0.5 kg using an electronic scale. For both measurements, participants wore light cloths and no shoes.

2.3. Integrative Neuromuscular Training Protocol

Participants returned to the Human Performance Laboratory to perform the INT protocol within 2 to 7 days of the peak aerobic capacity test. The INT protocol used in this study was based on previous pediatric research [11,14,15,27] and included strength- and skill-building exercises that were appropriate for children [10]. Our INT protocol consisted of the following six exercises: (1) balance board squats (EX1; 15 repetitions), (2) medicine ball squats with toss and catch (EX2; 15 repetitions), (3) BOSU™ planks with side steps (EX3; 20 repetitions), (4) medicine ball forward lunges (EX4; 16 repetitions), (5) battling rope double arm waves (EX5; 30 repetitions) and medicine balls slams (EX6; 15 repetitions). The 6 INT exercises were performed in successive order with each exercise interval lasting 30 s in duration. Each exercise was performed twice with a rest interval of 30 s in between sets and exercises. The 12 time intervals corresponding to the initiation and termination of each 30 s INT set were carefully monitored and labeled. The total duration of the INT protocol was 12 min (including 30 s recovery following the last exercise).

Pilot testing from our center found that a 2.3 kg medicine ball and a 4.1 kg battling rope were appropriate for children. Participants were asked to follow a specific cadence using a metronome and to try and complete a target number of repetitions during each set. A research assistant performed the INT protocol at the desired cadence with each participant during each set and provided a quick review of the upcoming exercise during each rest interval. All participants performed the same exercises in the same order. Participants were asked to manually indicate their RPE after each INT set on a visually presented scale consisting of verbal expressions with a numerical response range of 0 to 10 and five pictorial descriptors that represent a child at varying levels of exertion [26]. Participants became familiar with the INT protocol during a familiarization session which took place after the peak aerobic capacity test. During the familiarization session participants practiced each INT exercise and proper technique was reinforced with exercise-specific coaching cues.

2.4. Treadmill Protocol

Participants performed the TM trial 2 to 7 days after the INT protocol. The TM protocol used in this study was designed to be a moderate-intensity walking protocol that is consistent with general physical activity recommendations for school-age children [28,29]. Participants walked briskly at a predetermined exercise intensity of 50% VO$_2$ peak for 12 min. The speed and grade of the treadmill were adjusted to maintain the desired exercise intensity throughout the 12-min session. Cardiometabolic data were collected during the same 30 s time intervals as INT. Participants were asked to manually indicate their RPE during the TM trial [26].

2.5. Experimental Measurements: Oxygen Uptake and Heart Rate

VO_2 and HR were measured at rest and throughout the INT and TM protocols following similar experimental procedures. On arrival, each participant was asked to drink water *ad libitum* to prehydrate and was fitted with the same child-size respiratory mask and heart rate monitor used for the maximal aerobic capacity test. HR data were downloaded for analysis using a computer software program. HR data analyzed were the mean values collected during each 30-s time interval throughout the 12-min INT and TM protocols. Breath-by-breath VO_2 was measured during the INT and TM protocols using the same metabolic system used for maximal aerobic capacity testing. Values for relative VO_2, minute ventilation (V_E) and respiratory exchange ratio (RER) were recorded during the entire protocol. Individual breath-by-breath data points for all metabolic variables were averaged for each 30 s interval. Prior to each trial, each participant sat quietly in a chair for 5 min to collect baseline data. Once complete, the researcher briefly reviewed session instructions. Subsequently, each participant performed 2 to 3 min of calisthenics (e.g., arm circles and knee lifts) prior to INT or 2 to 3 min of low intensity walking prior to TM. Verbal encouragement was provided throughout the INT and TM trials.

2.6. Statistical Analysis

Descriptive statistics (mean ± SD) were calculated for all dependent variables. For each protocol, the mean values for VO_2, V_E, RER, and HR were averaged every 30 s in time-match intervals as well as for the entire 12-min protocol. A 2 (INT or TM) × 12 (time interval sets) analysis of variance with repeated measures was used to analyze within and between participant cardiometabolic and RPE data. A significant F ratio was followed by pairwise comparisons to detect differences between INT and TM at a given time interval using Bonferroni's adjustments. In addition, a dependent *t*-test was used to compare mean VO_2, V_E, RER, and HR of the entire protocol between INT and TM. For all statistical tests, a probability level of $p < 0.05$ denoted statistical significance. Statistical analyses were conducted in SPSS (version 24; SPSS, Chicago, IL, USA).

3. Results

All participants completed study procedures and no injuries or unexpected events occurred. Our post hoc comparisons revealed a progressive increase in cardiometabolic demand as VO_2, V_E, RER, and HR increased significantly throughout our multi-exercise INT protocol. During the INT protocol mean HR significantly increased from 121.1 ± 9.0 b·min^{-1} to 183.5 ± 7.9 b·min^{-1} and mean VO_2 significantly increased from 14.9 ± 3.6 mL·kg^{-1}·min^{-1} to 34.0 ± 6.4 mL·kg^{-1}·min^{-1} (Table 1). Values for HR, V_E, and RER tended to increase with each successive INT exercise and paralleled VO_2 data. Mean VO_2 and HR during EX5 and EX6 of the INT protocol were significantly higher than during time-matched TM intervals (Table 1) (all *Ps* < 0.05). Figure 1; Figure 2 depict the gradual increase in HR and VO_2, respectively, during the INT protocol as compared to TM.

Table 1. Cardiometabolic responses during integrative neuromuscular training (INT) and treadmill (TM) walking.

Interval (min)	INT EX/set	VO$_2$ INT	VO$_2$ TM	V$_E$ INT	V$_E$ TM	HR INT	HR TM	RER INT	RER TM
1 (0–0.5)	1/1	14.9 ± 3.6 [b-l]	19.2 ± 2.5	14.9 ± 4.5 [b-l]	16.8 ± 2.5	121.1 ± 9.0 [b-d,g-l]	121.1 ± 11.7	0.88 ± 0.07 [j-l]	0.82 ± 0.05
2 (1.0–1.5)	1/2	19.7 ± 3.9 [a,d,h-l]	23.4 ± 3.7	19.7 ± 6.6 [a,d,e,h-l]	20.8 ± 4.5	129.6 ± 10.9 [a,c-d,g-l]	133.8 ± 12.2	0.88 ± 0.08 [j-l]	0.85 ± 0.06
3 (2.0–2.5)	2/1	23.9 ± 8.2 [a,j-l]	25.4 ± 5.7	24.7 ± 7.7 [a,j-l]	23.8 ± 6.0	139.1 ± 11.6 [a,b,d,j-l]	139.3 ± 13.7	0.90 ± 0.07 [j-l]	0.89 ± 0.04
4 (3.0–3.5)	2/2	25.2 ± 6.3 [a,b,j-l]	25.8 ± 6.6	27.9 ± 9.2 [a,b,j-l]	24.2 ± 6.6	147.3 ± 12.4 [a-c,j-l]	146.0 ± 14.5	0.93 ± 0/07 [j-l]	0.90 ± 0.05
5 (4.0–4.5)	3/1	23.2 ± 4.7 [a,j-l]	26.6 ± 5.6	26.7 ± 9.5 [a,b,j-l]	25.4 ± 7.0	138.4 ± 19.0 [j-l]	145.1 ± 16.1	0.96 ± 0.07 [j-l]	0.90 ± 0.06
6 (5.0–5.5)	3/2	20.5 ± 4.3 [a,h-l]	26.4 ± 5.3 *	23.4 ± 9.4 [a,h-l]	25.0 ± 6.9	134.3 ± 16.5 [j-l]	148.1 ± 16.2	0.94 ± 0.06 [j-l]	0.90 ± 0.06
7 (6.0–6.5)	4/1	21.2 ± 3.4 [a,h-l]	27.2 ± 4.7 *	24.3 ± 9.1 [a,b,l]	25.8 ± 5.8	142.8 ± 13.6 [a,b,l]	150.0 ± 16.4	0.95 ± 0.07 [j-l]	0.90 ± 0.04
8 (7.0–7.5)	4/2	23.4 ± 4.2 [a,b,f,j-l]	27.5 ± 4.9 *	26.7 ± 9.1 [a,b,f,j-l]	26.6 ± 7.0	144.8 ± 14.0 [a,b,l]	150.1 ± 16.7	0.90 ± 0.05 [j-l]	0.90 ± 0.05
9 (8.0–8.5)	5/1	30.9 ± 9.1 [a,b,f,g]	27.8 ± 4.6	38.3 ± 14.2 [a-c,e-i]	26.7 ± 6.0	167.4 ± 10.5 [a-h,j-l]	151.1 ± 16.1	0.95 ± 0.08 [j-l]	0.91 ± 0.05
10 (9.0–9.5)	5/2	34.0 ± 6.4 [a-h]	27.6 ± 5.1 *	52.2 ± 12.4 [a-i]	26.4 ± 5.6 *	181.6 ± 8.3 [a-i, k,l]	151.3 ± 16.7 *	1.15 ± 0.07 [a-i]	0.90 ± 0.05 *
11 (10–10.5)	6/1	32.0 ± 5.4 [a-h]	27.6 ± 5.3 *	46.2 ± 10.2 [a-h]	26.7 ± 5.7 *	181.5 ± 9.0 [a-i]	150.5 ± 17.2 *	1.12 ± 0.07 [a-i]	0.90 ± 0.05 *
12 (11–11.5)	6/2	33.3 ± 6.0 [a-h]	26.8 ± 6.2 *	48.6 ± 11.0 [a-h]	25.1 ± 6.5 *	183.5 ± 7.9 [a-i]	150.4 ± 17.3 *	1.07 ± 0.06 [a-i]	0.89 ± 0.05 *

All values are mean ± SD. EX = exercise, VO$_2$ = oxygen uptake, mL·kg^{-1}·min^{-1}; V$_E$ = minute ventilation, L/min; HR = heart rate; RER = respiratory exchange ratio. [a] vs. interval 1; [b] vs. interval 2; [c] vs. interval 3; [d] vs. interval 4; [e] vs. interval 5; [f] vs. interval 6; [g] vs. interval 7; [h] vs. interval 8; [i] vs. interval 9; [j] vs. interval 10; [k] vs. interval 11; [l] vs. interval 12. * different than INT. $p \leq 0.05$.

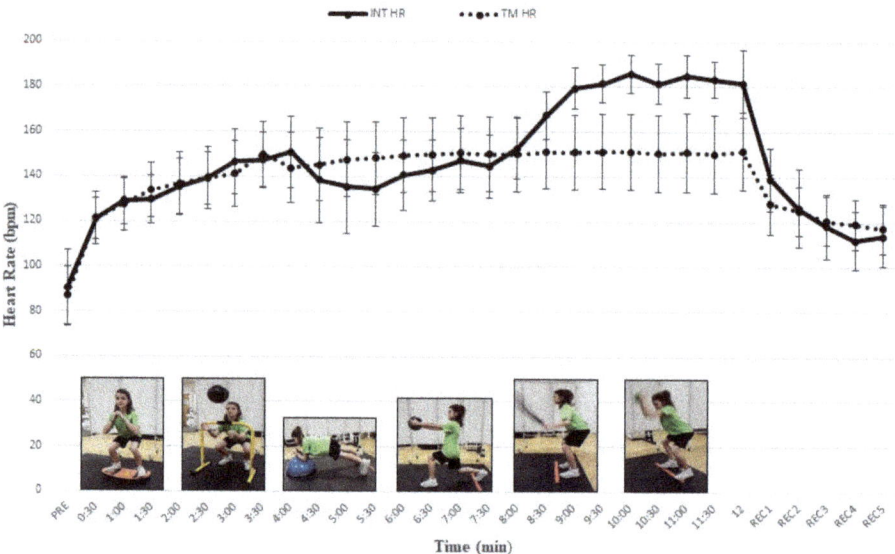

Figure 1. Heart rate (HR) responses (mean ± SD) during integrative neuromuscular training (INT) and treadmill (TM) protocols. PRE = Baseline; REC = recovery. See Table 1 for significant differences between INT exercises and protocols.

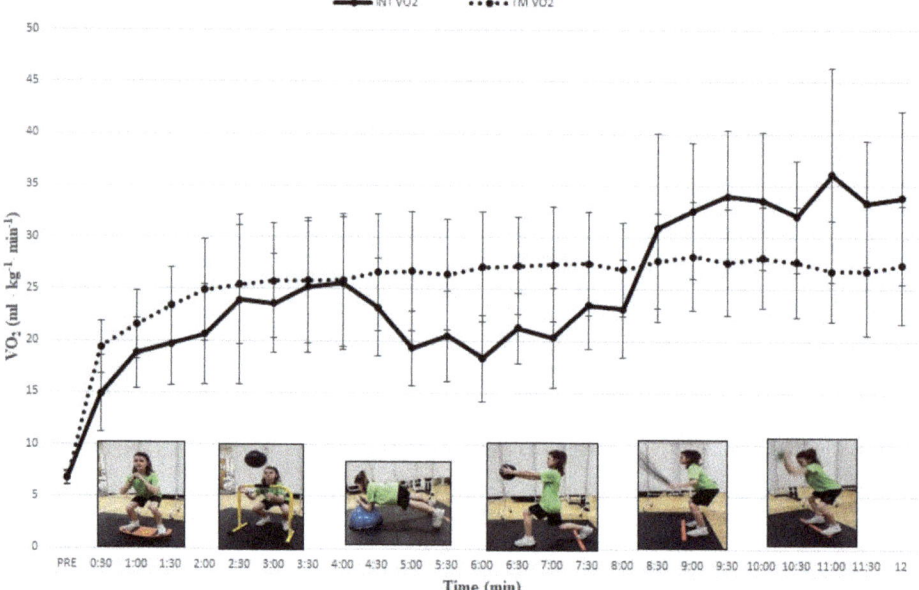

Figure 2. Relative oxygen uptake responses (mean ± SD) during integrative neuromuscular training (INT) and treadmill (TM) protocols. PRE = Baseline; See Table 1 for significant differences between INT exercises and protocols.

The relative cardiometabolic intensity of each INT exercise (expressed as a percentage of values attained during maximal aerobic capacity testing) ranged from 61.0% to 92.4% for HR and from 28.2% to 64.3% for VO_2. The relative cardiometabolic demands of each INT exercise compared to time-matched

TM time intervals are outlined on Table 2. The significant increases in cardiometabolic responses during INT mirrored significant increases in RPE. The mean RPEs (out of 10) for INT EX1 to EX6 were 1.14 ± 0.85, 2.26 ± 0.98, 2.91 ± 1.04, 3.55 ± 1.23, 5.42 ± 1.45 and 6.68 ± 1.67, respectively. There was no significant difference in mean VO_2 between the entire 12-min INT and TM protocols; however, mean values for HR, V_E and RER for the entire 12-min protocol were significantly higher during INT than TM (all $Ps < 0.05$) (Table 3). The mean VO_2 throughout the 12-min TM protocol was 49.5% of VO_2 peak attained during maximal aerobic capacity testing.

Table 2. Relative cardiometabolic intensity during integrative neuromuscular training (INT) and treadmill (TM) walking intervals.

Interval (min)	INT EX/Set	% VO_2 Peak		%HR Peak	
		INT	TM	INT	TM
1 (0–0.5)	1/1	28.2	36.3	61.0	61.0
2 (1.0–1.5)	1/2	37.2	44.2	65.3	67.4
3 (2.0–2.5)	2/1	45.1	48.0	70.1	70.1
4 (3.0–3.5)	2/2	47.6	48.8	74.2	73.5
5 (4.0–4.5)	3/1	43.8	50.2	69.7	73.1
6 (5.0–5.5)	3/2	38.7	49.9	67.6	74.6
7 (6.0–6.5)	4/1	40.0	51.4	71.9	75.6
8 (7.0–7.5)	4/2	44.2	52.0	72.9	75.6
9 (8.0–8.5)	5/1	58.4	52.5	84.3	76.1
10 (9.0–9.5)	5/2	64.3	52.2	91.5	76.2
11 (10–10.5)	6/1	60.5	52.2	91.4	75.8
12 (11–11.5)	6/2	62.9	50.7	92.4	75.8

Table 3. Mean cardiometabolic responses during the entire 12 min integrative neuromuscular training (INT) and treadmill (TM) protocols.

	INT	TM
VO_2 (mL·kg^{-1}·min^{-1})	25.4 ± 4.5	26.2 ± 4.5
V_E (l·min^{-1})	29.79 ± 8.0	24.7 ± 5.5 *
HR (beats·min^{-1})	153.4 ± 10.6	145.2 ± 15.0 *
RER	0.96 ± 0.04	0.89 ± 0.05 *

All values are mean ± SD. * different than INT. $p \leq 0.05$.

4. Discussion

The aim of our study was to examine the acute cardiometabolic responses to a multi-modal INT protocol in children and to compare these responses to a bout of moderate-intensity TM walking. Consistent with our hypothesis, we found a progressive, multi-modal INT protocol comprising 30 s of work with 30 s of passive recovery can pose a moderate to vigorous cardiometabolic stimulus in children and selected INT exercises can be equal to or more metabolically challenging than TM walking. While other pediatric investigations detailed the acute physiological responses to intermittent bouts of single-mode exercise with cycling, sprinting, medicine balls or battling ropes [14,15,30,31], this is the first study to describe the acute cardiometabolic demands of a mixed-exercise INT protocol in children. No significant differences were observed in mean VO_2 between the entire 12-min INT and TM protocols. However, mean HR, V_E, and RER were significantly higher during INT than TM. Given the link between vigorous physical activity and positive health outcomes in youth [17–19], our findings provide insight into the potential cardiometabolic benefits of INT if performed at the requisite weekly frequency.

Participants in our study were physically active children with a peak aerobic capacity of 52.9 ± 9.4 mL·kg^{-1}·min^{-1} and a peak HR of 198.5 ± 5.5 bpm. During the INT protocol, VO_2 increased from 14.9 ± 3.6 to 34.0 ± 6.4 mL·kg^{-1}·min^{-1} and HR increased from 121.1 ± 9.0 bpm to 183.5 ± 7.9 bpm (Table 1). As shown on Table 2, the relative intensity of each INT exercise expressed as a percentage of VO_2 peak and HR peak ranged from 28.2% to 64.3% and from 61.0% to 92.4%, respectively. The mean VO_2 and HR responses during the entire 12 min INT protocol were 49.5% and 73.1%, respectively, of peak values. When compared to a standard classification of physical activity intensity based on percentage of VO_2 peak or HR peak, our findings indicate that the overall intensity of our 12-min INT protocol could be characterized as "moderate" (i.e., 46–63% VO_2 peak and 64–76% HR peak) whereas the intensity of individual INT exercises could be characterized as "light", "moderate", or "vigorous" depending upon the mode and complexity of each movement [32]. Knowing the intensity levels of different INT exercises can help researchers and practitioners design interventions that optimize training-induced adaptations and encourage compliance in all participants.

The progressive increase in HR throughout our INT protocol was consistent with other reports that examined the acute physiological responses to different modes of resistance exercise in youth [14,15,20]. During a 10-min bout of medicine ball interval training (30 s/exercise and 30 s rest/set) researchers reported that mean HR values during work sets ranged from 121.5 ± 12.3 bpm (61.1% HR peak) to 178.3 ± 9.4 bpm (89.6% HR peak) [14]. Harris and colleagues characterized the acute responses to resistance exercise and HIIT in early adolescents (12–13 years) and reported mean HR over all 12 work sets of 169.9 ± 9.2 bpm for resistance training and 179.0 ± 5.6 bpm for HIIT which represented 85% and 90% of HR peak, respectively [20]. In our study, the gradual increase in HR from 61% HR peak to over 90% HR peak was expected because the structure of our multi-modal INT protocol included six different exercises that progressed from a less intense squatting exercise to a more explosive movement. These findings are notable because high-intensity interval training characterized by short bouts of vigorous intensity activity may be needed to elicit the greatest improvements in cardiometabolic health and aerobic fitness in children [21,33]. Of interest, participants in our study recovered quickly from the demands of INT as evidenced by heart rates of 139.1 ± 13.9 bpm, 118.4 ± 14.2 bpm, and 113.9 ± 13.5 bpm after 1, 3 and 5 min of recovery, respectively (Figure 2). These observations are consistent with others who reported a faster post-exercise recovery heart rate in children than endurance adult athletes. [34].

The findings related to relative VO_2, V_E and RER build upon previous reports investigating different modes of youth resistance training. During a progressive interval protocol with 5 battling rope exercises, relative VO_2, V_E and RER increased to 30.0 mL·kg^{-1}·min^{-1} (64.8% VO_2 peak), 40.8 L/min and 1.07, respectively [15]. In another report, relative VO_2, V_E and RER reached 34.9 mL·kg^{-1}·min^{-1} (63.6% VO_2 peak), 40.4 L/min and 0.95, respectively, during medicine ball interval training [14]. While Baquet and colleagues reported mean VO_2 values of 35.5 mL·kg^{-1}·min^{-1} (64.6% VO_2 peak) to 47.0 mL·kg^{-1}·min^{-1} (85.9% VO_2 peak) during sprint high intensity interval exercise in children [31], differences in exercise characteristics, workload duration and rest interval length can explain, at least in part, these findings. The progressive increase in RER that reached values above 1.0 which were greater than those observed during TM walking further attested to the intense nature of our INT protocol. Collectively, it appears that INT and other types of interval training could be used to bring about positive cardiometabolic adaptations in children.

Our findings demonstrate that INT characterized by short exercise intervals interspersed with brief rest intervals can pose a moderate to vigorous cardiometabolic stimulus in youth. Unlike brisk walking, INT typically requires the whole body to function as a unit in order to perform movements proficiently with proper technique at the desired cadence. During our multi-modal INT protocol, the highest VO_2 and HR values were achieved during EX5 (battling rope double arm wave) and EX6 (medicine ball slams), respectively. Both of these exercises require a substantial involvement of the upper and lower body since participants vigorously waved a 4.1 kg battling rope with both arms or forcibly slammed a 2.3 kg medicine ball against the floor at maximal or near maximal velocity. Interestingly, Ratamess and colleagues examined the acute cardiometabolic response to 13 different resistance exercise protocols in adults and found that the battling rope double arm wave elicited the highest responses [35]. While the greater complexity and muscle mass activation of the INT exercises towards the end of our protocol suggest that the choice of exercise is a primary determinant of the cardiometabolic responses to INT, the cumulative effects of fatigue and cardiovascular drift during our INT protocol should also be considered because the cardiometabolic responses to each INT exercise were likely influenced by the subsequent fatigue from the previous exercise.

The structure of our INT protocol was based on previous fitness interventions with children and included 2 sets of 6 different exercises with a 30 s rest interval in between sets and exercises [11,27]. Due to the age of the participants and the relative intensity of selected INT exercises, a progressive, multi-modal INT protocol with passive recovery intervals was arguably required to maintain safety, motivation and adherence. Sustained bouts (>10 min) of physical activity are rare in children and the natural tempo of their activity is characterized by short bursts lasting a few seconds [36]. Furthermore, it is important to note that the objective of our investigation was not to disentangle the acute demands of each INT exercise, but rather to examine the acute cardiometabolic responses to a novel INT protocol and to compare these responses to a more traditional form of continuous physical activity of comparable time and overall VO_2. Notably, we used a time period of 12 min so that the protocol could be readily incorporated into a physical education class or sports practice. With that said, the results from our investigation provide preliminary cardiometabolic reference values for a multi-modal INT protocol and highlight the versatility of INT because different exercises could be combined to offer light, moderate, vigorous or variable intensity training depending on the needs, goals and abilities of the children.

Our findings support the integration of INT into school- and community-based youth fitness programs and inform the development of interventions aimed at increasing time spent in MVPA. The progressive increase in cardiometabolic intensity throughout the INT protocol was consistent with the participants perceptions as evidenced by significant increases in RPE. Others found that youth could rate their perceived exertion during resistance training and our observations support the use of RPE to monitor the intensity of INT in children [20,37]. We also observed that our INT protocol was challenging and appealing for the participants. This was evidenced by 100% compliance with research instructions and testing protocols. Although the affective response to INT were not explored in our investigation, Malik and colleagues found that enjoyment was higher following high-intensity interval exercise compared with continuous moderate-intensity exercise in adolescents [38]. Given that a child's level of enjoyment is a strong predictor of physical activity participation [39], further examination of the affective responses to INT are warranted.

The INT exercises used in our investigation were intended to progress from less intense to more intense. EX1 consisted of squatting on a balance board at a controlled cadence and EX6 required participants to repeatedly slam a 2.3 kg medicine ball against the floor with energy and vigor. These are important considerations when discussing our findings because the cardiometabolic responses to INT are dependent upon various factors including the intensity of muscle actions, type of muscle actions, the amount of muscle mass used, rest intervals and body position [14,15,40]. In addition, age, fitness level and body mass index can influence the acute cardiometabolic responses to exercise and the kinetics of recovery after exercise [25,34,41]. Children appear to be less susceptible to neuromuscular fatigue than adults following resistance training [42] and the post-exercise decline in VO_2 seems to be faster in children with a higher peak VO_2 than those with a lower peak VO_2 [34,43]. Thus, the results of our investigation should be interpreted within the context of a mixed model exercise approach that reflects how children may actually perform INT during physical education or sports practice.

We acknowledge that the maturity status of the participants was not assessed and therefore we were unable to determine if all participants were prepubertal. Also, the participants in our study were active, healthy girls and boys so the homogeneity of our sample limits generalizability to other populations including those with illnesses or disabilities that alter movement or mechanical efficiency. It is also important to consider the design of our INT protocol and the limited INT experience of our participants. Acute program variables will impact the cardiometabolic responses to INT and as children become more skilled and efficient at performing INT exercises the acute cardiometabolic demands to a given protocol will not be constant. While other pediatric researchers examined the acute cardiometabolic responses to single-mode exercise, the design of our progressive, multi-modal INT protocol arguably provides greater translatability to school- and community-based programs in which the physical fitness levels and activity interests of children can vary widely.

5. Conclusions

INT has been investigated as a potentially potent and time efficient method of enhancing neuromuscular fitness in youth [11,12,16] and our novel findings suggest that this innovative training method consisting of strength- and skill-building exercises could also provide a sufficient training stimulus needed to induce cardiometabolic adaptations. Considering the amount of time children spend in MVPA during physical education and youth sport practice is falling short of expectations [44,45], INT could be a worthwhile addition to school- and community-based programs to target exercise deficits. Unlike continuous bouts of moderate-intensity walking, a progressive INT intervention with battling rope and medicine ball exercises may better prepare youth for the vigorous intensity nature of game and sport activities. These observations have practical relevance for teachers, coaches and health care providers who design exercise programs and sport practices for children. Altogether, the acute cardiometabolic responses to INT along with high compliance to our study procedures provide support for future training studies to better understand the multidimensional benefits of INT on health, fitness and performance in youth.

Author Contributions: Conceptualization, A.D.F., J.K. and N.A.R.; Formal analysis, A.D.F., J.K., N.A.R. and J.B.; Investigation, A.D.F., J.K., A.C.F., M.B., S.D. and C.J.; Methodology, A.D.F., J.K., M.B., S.D. and C.J.; Resources, A.D.F., J.K., N.A.R., A.C.F. and J.B.; Supervision, A.D.F., J.K. and A.C.F.; Writing—original draft, A.D.F. and J.K.; Writing—review & editing, A.D.F., J.K., N.A.R., A.C.F., M.B., S.D., C.J. and J.B.

Funding: This research received no external funding.

Conflicts of Interest: The authors declare no conflict of interest.

References

1. Aubert, S.; Barnes, J.; Abdeta, C.; Abi Nader, P.; Adeniyi, A.; Aguilar-Farias, N.; Andrade Tenesaca, D.; Bhawra, J.; Brazo-Sayavera, J.; Cardon, G.; et al. Global Matrix 3.0 Physical Activity Report Card Grades for Children and Youth: Results and Analysis From 49 Countries. *J. Phys. Act. Health* **2018**, *15*, S251–S273. [CrossRef] [PubMed]
2. Faigenbaum, A.; Rial Rebullido, T.; MacDonald, J. The unsolved problem of paediatric physical inactivity: It is time for a new perspective. *Acta Paediatr.* **2018**, *107*, 1857–1859. [CrossRef] [PubMed]

3. Metcalf, B.; Henley, W.; Wilkin, T. Effectiveness of intervention on physical activity of children: Systematic review and meta-analysis of controlled trials with objectively measured outcomes (EarlyBird 54). *BMJ* **2012**, *345*, e5888. [CrossRef] [PubMed]
4. Carlin, A.; Murphy, M.; Nevill, A.; Gallagher, A. Effects of a peer-led Walking In ScHools intervention (the WISH study) on physical activity levels of adolescent girls: a cluster randomised pilot study. *Trials* **2018**, *19*, 31. [CrossRef] [PubMed]
5. Villa-González, E.; Ruiz, J.; Mendoza, J.; Chillón, P. Effects of a school-based intervention on active commuting to school and health-related fitness. *BMC Public Health* **2017**, *17*, 20. [CrossRef] [PubMed]
6. Ruiz-Hermosa, A.; Martínez-Vizcaíno, V.; Alvarez-Bueno, C.; García-Prieto, J.; Pardo-Guijarro, M.; Sánchez-López, M. No association between active commuting to school, adiposity, fitness, and cognition in Spanish children: The MOVI-KIDS Study. *J. Sch. Health* **2018**, *88*, 836–846. [CrossRef] [PubMed]
7. Sandercock, G.; Cohen, D. Temporal trends in muscular fitness of English 10-year-olds 1998–2014: An allometric approach. *J. Sci. Med. Sport* **2019**, *22*, 201–205. [CrossRef] [PubMed]
8. Fraser, B.; Blizzard, L.; Tomkinson, G.; Lycett, K.; Wake, M.; Burgner, D.; Ranganathan, S.; Juonala, M.; Dwyer, T.; Venn, A.; et al. The great leap backward: changes in the jumping performance of Australian children aged 11-12-years between 1985 and 2015. *J. Sports Sci.* **2019**, *37*, 748–754. [CrossRef]
9. Smith, J.; Eather, N.; Weaver, R.; Riley, N.; Beets, M.; Lubans, D. Behavioral correlates of muscular fitness in children and adolescents: A systematic review. *Sports Med.* **2019**. epub ahead of print. [CrossRef]
10. Myer, G.; Faigenbaum, A.; Ford, K.; Best, T.; Bergeron, M.; Hewett, T. When to initiate integrative neuromuscular training to reduce sports-related injuries and enhance health in youth? *Curr. Sports Med. Rep.* **2011**, *10*, 155–166. [CrossRef]
11. Faigenbaum, A.; Farrell, A.; Fabiano, M.; Radler, T.; Naclerio, F.; Ratamess, N.; Kang, J.; Myer, G. Effects of integrated neuromuscular training on fitness performance in children. *Pediatr. Exerc. Sci.* **2011**, *23*, 573–584. [CrossRef]
12. Duncan, M.; Eyre, E.; Oxford, S. The effects of 10 weeks Integrated Neuromuscular Training on fundamental movement skills and physical self-efficacy in 6–7 year old children. *J. Strength Cond. Res.* **2018**, *32*, 3348–3356. [CrossRef] [PubMed]
13. Foss, K.; Thomas, S.; Khoury, J.; Myer, G.; Hewett, T. A school-based neuromuscular training program and sport-related injury incidence: A prospective randomized controlled clinical trial. *J. Athl. Train.* **2018**, *53*, 20–28. [CrossRef] [PubMed]
14. Faigenbaum, A.; Kang, J.; Ratamess, N.; Farrell, A.; Ellis, N.; Vought, I.; Bush, J. Acute cardiometabolic responses to medicine ball interval training in children. *Int. J. Exerc. Sci.* **2018**, *11*, 886–899. [PubMed]
15. Faigenbaum, A.; Kang, J.; Ratamess, N.; Farrell, A.; Golda, S.; Stranieri, A.; Coe, J.; Bush, J. Acute cardiometabolic responses to battling rope exercise in children. *J. Strength Cond. Res.* **2018**, *32*, 1197–1206. [CrossRef] [PubMed]
16. Panagoulis, C.; Chatzinikolaou, A.; Avloniti, A.; Leontsini, D.; Deli, C.; Draganidis, D.; Stampoulis, T.; Oikonomou, T.; Papanikolaou, K.; Rafailakis, L.; et al. In-season integrative neuromuscular strength training improves performance of early adolescent soccer athletes. *J. Strength Cond. Res.* **2018**. epub before print. [CrossRef]
17. Tarp, J.; Child, A.; White, T.; Westgate, K.; Bugge, A.; Grøntved, A.; Wedderkopp, N.; Andersen, L.; Cardon, G.; Davey, R.; et al. Physical activity intensity, bout-duration, and cardiometabolic risk markers in children and adolescents. *Int. J. Obes. (Lond.)* **2018**, *42*, 1639–1650. [CrossRef]
18. Aadland, E.; Andersen, L.; Anderssen, S.; Resaland, G.; Kvalheim, O. Associations of volumes and patterns of physical activity with metabolic health in children: A multivariate pattern analysis approach. *Prev. Med.* **2018**, *115*, 12–18. [CrossRef]
19. Hamer, M.; Stamatakis, E. Relative proportion of vigorous physical activity, total volume of moderate to vigorous activity, and body mass index in youth: the Millennium Cohort Study. *Int. J. Obes. (Lond.)* **2018**, *42*, 1239–1242. [CrossRef]
20. Harris, N.; Dulson, D.; Logan, G.; Warbrick, I.; Merien, F.; Lubans, D. Acute responses to resistance and high-intensity interval training in early adolescents. *J. Strength Cond. Res.* **2016**, *31*, 1177–1186. [CrossRef]
21. Bond, B.; Weston, K.; Williams, C.; Barker, A. Perspectives on high-intensity interval exercise for health promotion in children and adolescents. *Open Access J. Sports Med.* **2017**, *8*, 243–265. [CrossRef] [PubMed]

22. Thivel, D.; Masurier, J.; Baquet, G.; Timmons, B.; Pereira, B.; Berthoin, S.; Duclos, M.; Aucouturier, J. High-intensity interval training in overweight and obese children and adolescents: systematic review and meta-analysis. *J. Sports Med. Phys. Fitness* **2019**, *59*, 310–324. [CrossRef] [PubMed]
23. Institute of Medicine. *Educating the Student Body: Taking Physical Activity and Physical Education to School*; The National Academies Press: Washington, DC, USA, 2013.
24. Kotte, E.; DE Groot, J.; Bongers, B.; Winkler, A.; Takken, T. Validity and reproducibility of a new treadmill protocol: The fitkids treadmill test. *Med. Sci. Sports Exerc.* **2015**, *47*, 2241–2247. [CrossRef]
25. Armstrong, N.; McManus, A. Aerobic Fitness. In *Oxford Textbook of Children's Sport and Exercise Medicine*, 3rd ed.; Armstrong, N., van Mechelen, W., Eds.; Oxford University Press: Oxford, UK, 2017; pp. 161–180.
26. Faigenbaum, A.D.; Milliken, L.A.; Cloutier, G.; Westcott, W.L. Perceived exertion during resistance exercise by children. *Percept. Mot. Skills* **2004**, *98*, 627–637. [CrossRef]
27. Faigenbaum, A.; Bush, J.; McLoone, R.; Kreckel, M.; Farrell, A.; Ratamess, N.; Kang, J. Benefits of strength and skill-based training during primary school physical education. *J. Strength Cond. Res.* **2015**, *29*, 1255–1262. [CrossRef]
28. U.S. Department of Health and Human Services. *Physical Activity Guidelines for Americans*; U.S. Department of Health and Human Services: Washington, DC, USA, 2018; p. 49.
29. Butte, N.; Watson, K.; Ridle, Y.K.; Zakeri, I.; McMurray, R.; Pfeiffer, K.; Crouter, S.; Herrmann, S.; Bassett, D.; Long, A.; et al. A Youth Compendium of Physical Activities: Activity Codes and Metabolic Intensities. *Med. Sci. Sports Exerc.* **2018**, *50*, 246–256. [CrossRef]
30. Chuensiri, N.; Tanaka, H.; Suksom, D. The acute effects of supramaximal high-intensity intermittent exercise on vascular function in lean vs. obese prepubescent boys. *Pediatr. Exerc. Sci.* **2015**, *27*, 503–509. [CrossRef] [PubMed]
31. Baquet, G.; Gamelin, F.; Aucouturier, J.; Berthoin, S. Cardiorespiratory responses to continuous and intermittent exercise in children. *Int. J. Sports Med.* **2017**, *38*, 755–762. [CrossRef]
32. American College of Sports Medicine. *ACSM's Guidelines for Exercise Testing and Prescription*, 10th ed.; Lippincott, Williams and Wilkins: Baltimore, MD, USA, 2018.
33. Eddolls, W.; McNarry, M.; Stratton, G.; Winn, C.; Mackintosh, K. High-intensity interval training interventions in children and adolescents: A systematic review. *Sports Med.* **2017**, *47*, 2326–2374. [CrossRef]
34. Birat, A.; Bourdier, P.; Piponnier, E.; Blazevich, A.; Maciejewski, H.; Duché, P.; Ratel, S. Metabolic and fatigue profiles are comparable between prepubertal children and well-trained adult endurance athletes. *Front. Pediatr.* **2018**, *9*, 387. [CrossRef]
35. Ratamess, N.; Rosenberg, J.; Klei, S.; Dougherty, B.; Kang, J.; Smith, C.; Ross, R.; Faigenbaum, A. Comparison of the acute metabolic responses to traditional resistance, body-weight, and battling rope exercise. *J. Strength Cond. Res.* **2015**, *29*, 47–57. [CrossRef]
36. Riddoch, C.; Mattocks, C.; Deere, K.; Saunders, J.; Kirkby, J.; Tilling, K.; Leary, S.; Blair, S.; Ness, A. Objective measurement of levels and patterns of physical activity. *Arch. Dis. Childhood* **2007**, *92*, 963–969. [CrossRef]
37. Robertson, R.; Goss, F.; Aaron, D.; Nagle, E.; Gallagher, M.; Kane, I.; Tessmer, K.; Schafer, M.; Hunt, S. Concurrent muscle hurt and perceived exertion of children during resistance exercise. *Med. Sci. Sports Exerc.* **2009**, *41*, 1146–1154. [CrossRef]
38. Malik, A.; Williams, C.; Bond, B.; Weston, K.; Barker, A. Acute cardiorespiratory, perceptual and enjoyment responses to high-intensity interval exercise in adolescents. *Eur. J. Sport Sci.* **2017**, *17*, 1335–1342. [CrossRef]
39. Sebire, S.; Jago, R.; Fox, K.; Edwards, M.; Thompson, J. Testing a self-determination theory model of children's physical activity motivation: a cross-sectional study. *Int. J. Behav. Nutr. Phys. Act.* **2013**, *10*, 111. [CrossRef]
40. Ratamess, N. *ACSM's Foundations of Strength Training and Conditioning*; Lippincott, Williams and Wilkins: Philadelphia, PA, USA, 2012.
41. Nikolaidis, P.; Kintziou, E.; Georgoudis, G.; Afonso, J.; Vancini, R.; Knechtle, B. The effect of body mass index on acute cardiometabolic responses to graded exercise testing in children: A narrative review. *Sports* **2018**, *6*, 103. [CrossRef]
42. Murphy, J.; Button, D.; Chaouachi, A.; Behm, D. Prepubescent males are less susceptible to neuromuscular fatigue following resistance exercise. *Eur. J. Appl. Physiol.* **2014**, *114*, 825–835. [CrossRef]
43. Singh, T.; Alexander, M.; Gauvreau, K.; Curran, T.; Rhodes, Y.; Rhodes, J. Recovery of oxygen consumption after maximal exercise in children. *Med. Sci. Sports Exerc.* **2011**, *43*, 555–559. [CrossRef]

44. Hollis, J.; Williams, A.; Sutherland, R.; Campbell, E.; Nathan, N.; Wolfenden, L.; Morgan, P.; Lubans, D.; Wiggers, J. A systematic review and meta-analysis of moderate-to-vigorous physical activity levels in elementary school physical education lessons. *Prev. Med.* **2016**, *86*, 34–54. [CrossRef]
45. Schlechter, C.; Rosenkranz, R.; Milliken, G.; Dzewaltowski, D. Physical activity levels during youth sport practice: Does coach training or experience have an influence? *J. Sports Sci.* **2017**, *35*, 22–28. [CrossRef]

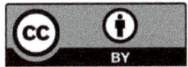

© 2019 by the authors. Licensee MDPI, Basel, Switzerland. This article is an open access article distributed under the terms and conditions of the Creative Commons Attribution (CC BY) license (http://creativecommons.org/licenses/by/4.0/).

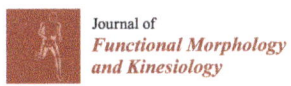

Article

Validation of Cardiorespiratory Fitness Measurements in Adolescents

Pedro Migliano [1], Laura S. Kabiri [2], Megan Cross [1], Allison Butcher [1], Amy Frugé [1], Wayne Brewer [1] and Alexis Ortiz [3,*]

1 School of Physical Therapy, Texas Woman's University, 6700 Fannin, Houston, TX 77030, USA
2 Department of Kinesiology, Rice University, 6100 Main Street, Houston, TX 77005, USA
3 Department of Physical Therapy, UT Health San Antonio, 7703 Floyd Curl Dr. San Antonio, TX 78229, USA
* Correspondence: ortiza7@uthscsa.edu; Tel.: +1-210-567-8750; Fax: +1-210-567-8774

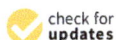

Received: 28 June 2019; Accepted: 11 July 2019; Published: 13 July 2019

Abstract: Cardiorespiratory fitness (CRF) is an important indicator of adolescent cardiovascular well-being and future cardiometabolic health but not always feasible to measure. The purpose of this study was to estimate the concurrent validity of the non-exercise test (NET) for adolescents against the Progressive Aerobic Capacity Endurance Run (PACER®) and direct measures of VO_{2max} as well as to examine the concurrent validity of the PACER® with a portable metabolic system (K4b²™). Forty-six adolescents (12–17 years) completed the NET prior to performing the PACER® while wearing the K4b²™. The obtained VO_{2max} values were compared using linear regression, intra-class correlation (ICC), and Bland–Altman plots, and α was set at 0.05. The VO_{2max} acquired directly from the K4b²™ was significantly correlated to the VO_{2max} indirectly estimated from the NET ($r = 0.73$, $p < 0.001$, $r^2 = 0.53$, ICC = 0.67). PACER® results were significantly related to the VO_{2max} estimates from the NET ($r = 0.81$, $p < 0.001$, $r^2 = 0.65$, ICC = 0.72). Direct measures from the K4b²™ were significantly correlated to the VO_{2max} estimates from the PACER® ($r = 0.87$, $p < 0.001$, $r^2 = 0.75$, ICC = 0.93). The NET is a valid measure of CRF in adolescents and can be used when an exercise test is not feasible.

Keywords: VO_{2max}; PACER; non-exercise test

1. Introduction

Low cardiorespiratory fitness (CRF) levels in adolescents have been linked to insulin resistance as well as cardiovascular and cardiometabolic risk factors [1–5]. Higher levels of CRF in adolescents have also been linked to improved academic outcomes and an improved ability to regulate attention and behavior [6,7]. There is a strong positive relationship between CRF and cognitive performance, with multiple studies showing that adolescents with higher levels of CRF outperformed their peers with lower levels of CRF in cognitive tests involving working memory, cognitive flexibility, and inhibition, which is the ability to ignore extraneous environmental information [8–10]. The improved cognitive ability is thought to be due to the increased volume in different regions of the brain such as the hippocampus and basal ganglia found in adolescents with higher levels of CRF [8,11]. Moreover, higher CRF has been shown to be an excellent predictor of physical activity level during adulthood [12,13]. Since CRF is an important health predictor in adolescents, it should be regularly assessed in both healthcare and school settings.

Maximal oxygen uptake (VO_{2max}), expressed as mL/kg/min of oxygen, is the gold standard measure of CRF and can be measured both directly and indirectly [14,15]. A direct measure of VO_{2max} is obtained by ventilatory gas analysis during a graded exercise test at maximum exertion and is the most precise measure of VO_{2max} [14]. An indirect measure estimates VO_{2max} from a maximal or submaximal exercise test and is usually estimated from total time, total work, or heart rate [15]. Especially in school settings, VO_{2max} is often indirectly measured and estimated using a field test. While there are a few different options when it comes to field tests to indirectly measure VO_{2max}, the 20-m multistage shuttle run test (20MSR) is the most frequently used test, as it has shown moderate to high criterion validity compared to direct measures of VO_{2max} and is a more practical test compared to longer duration endurance tests, such as the 6-min endurance run [16,17]. The Progressive Aerobic Cardiovascular Endurance Run (PACER®) is part of the FitnessGram® tests administered to adolescents in schools [18]. The PACER® is a 20MSR meant to mimic a maximal exertion exercise test with workloads increasing every stage until the participant reaches volitional exhaustion. The standardized procedure of the PACER® has participants run between two markers placed 20 m apart while keeping pace to a prerecorded audio cadence that increases every minute. The test is terminated if a participant fails to reach a marker for the second time or if the participant can no longer continue. This field test has been shown to be both reliable (intra-class correlation (ICC): 0.77–0.93) and valid (r: 0.62–0.83) [16,19,20], when compared to directly measured VO_{2max} during a treadmill maximal exercise test.

It is not always possible to directly assess VO_{2max} in all settings, such as schools, gyms, or even in a clinical setting. Ventilatory gas analysis is time-consuming and requires expensive equipment that prevents the mass screening which would be required in a school setting or in the daily caseload and time restraints of a healthcare professional. The non-exercise test (NET) is a paper-based questionnaire used to estimate VO_{2max} from different variables including sex, age, body mass index (BMI), resting heart rate, and self-reported habitual physical activity levels [21,22]. Use of this questionnaire allows for both quick and widespread CRF screening without any health risk to the participants. The NET has been shown to be valid within the adult population [21], but to the best of our knowledge, has not been tested within the adolescent population. Therefore, the purpose of this study was to estimate the concurrent validity of the NET for adolescents against the PACER® test and objective measures of VO_{2max} as well as to examine the concurrent validity of the VO_{2max} estimated by the PACER® with the VO_{2max} obtained from the Cosmed K4b^{2TM} portable metabolic system (Cosmed K4b^2, Cosmed, Rome, Italy) during the PACER® test.

2. Materials and Methods

2.1. Subjects

Adolescents aged 12–17 years were recruited by email, education support groups, co-operatives, and word of mouth. Parents were asked if their child had any physical or mental limitations that would prevent them from safely and accurately completing the test and if any were noted, the child was excluded. Institutional review board approval (Protocol #19736 on 19 January 2017) from Texas Woman's University in Houston, TX, parental informed consent, and minor assent were secured prior to any subject enrollment or data collection.

2.2. Procedures

Height and weight were assessed barefoot with light clothing using a medical-grade stadiometer calibrated prior to its use. Pubertal level was assessed using the pubertal developmental scale.

Prior to participating in the PACER and being fitted with the K4b^{2TM}, participants were given the NET questionnaire previously validated in adults by Jurca et al. [21]. As required by the NET, each participant was asked to choose the physical activity level which best described their daily level of activity, as listed in Table 1. Participant BMI was calculated based on their weight and height measurement. Resting heart rate (RHR) was measured with the SantaMedical SM150BL finger pulse oximeter (SantaMedical, Tustin, CA, USA) as the final measurement after sitting for at least five minutes.

Table 1. Physical Activity Levels for NET.

Physical Activity Level	Description	Score
1	Inactive or little activity other than usual daily activities.	0.00
2	Regularly (≥5 d/wk) participate in physical activities requiring low levels of exertion that result in slight increases in breathing and heart rate for at least 10 min at a time.	0.32
3	Participate in aerobic exercises such as brisk walking, jogging or running, cycling, swimming, or vigorous sports at a comfortable pace or other activities requiring similar levels of exertion for 20 to 60 min per week.	1.06
4	Participate in aerobic exercises such as brisk walking, jogging or running at a comfortable pace, or other activities requiring similar levels of exertion for 1 to 3 h per week.	1.76
5	Participate in aerobic exercises such as brisk walking, jogging or running at a comfortable pace, or other activities requiring similar levels of exertion for over 3 h per week.	3.03

NET equation: $VO_{2max} = 3.5 * ((Sex * 2.77) - (age * 0.1) - (BMI * 0.17) - (RHR * 0.03) + (physical\ activity\ score * 1.00) + 18.07)$; Sex: 0 = F, 1 = M.

The K4b2^{TM} portable metabolic system was used to directly measure VO_{2max} during the PACER®. The K4b2^{TM} has demonstrated high test–retest reliability (ICC = 0.70–0.90) [23] and has shown to be valid in VO_2 measurement when compared to a traditional stationary gas exchange system (r: 0.93–0.97) [24]. The K4b2^{TM} was calibrated according to manufacturer's recommendations using known gases and room air sampling. After calibration, participants were fitted with a mask and connected to the K4b2^{TM} prior to initiating the PACER®.

After donning the K4b2^{TM}, adolescents were allowed to wear and familiarize themselves with the device for 5 min. Participants completed the 20-m PACER® individually as per the standardized instructions. Two pieces of tape were placed 20 m apart, denoting the crossing lines for the PACER®, and the FitnessGram® cadence soundtrack was played at a volume loud enough for the participant to hear. Participants were instructed to begin running when they heard the first beep on the soundtrack. For the lap to be valid, each participant was required to clear at least one foot over the line prior to the next beep. The test was terminated following the second miss or if the participant desired to stop. All raters were trained and followed the standardized test procedures. Once the PACER® had been terminated, total laps were recorded, the K4b2^{TM} data was saved, and the mask was doffed.

VO_{2max} with the K4b2^{TM} system was determined in the same manner used by Silva et al. [25]. Respiratory variables were recorded breath-by-breath and averaged over a 10-s period. VO_{2max} was determined when a plateau in the VO_2 curve was detected and if the plateau was absent the VO_{2peak} was taken instead. VO_{2max} with the PACER® was calculated using the quadratic model established by Mahar, Guerieri, Hanna, and Kemble [26]: $VO_{2max} = 41.76799 + (0.49261 \times laps) - (0.00290 \times laps^2) - (0.61613 \times BMI) + (0.34787 \times sex \times age)$, where sex is 0 for males and 1 for females.

2.3. Statistical Analyses

The Shapiro–Wilk test, Levene's test, and box plots were utilized to screen all data for normality assumptions, homoscedasticity, and outliers, respectively. Linear regressions with Pearson correlations were performed on the VO_{2max} estimates acquired from the PACER® and the NET, and the VO_{2max} acquired from the K4b2^{TM} system. Intra-class correlations (ICCs), standard error of estimate (SEE), paired sample t-tests, and Bland–Altman plots were performed to assess agreement and differences between the measures of VO_{2max}. All statistical analyses were conducted with IBM SPSS software for Windows (v. 25.0; IBM Corp., Armonk, NY, USA).

3. Results

Forty-six adolescents (male: 24; female: 22) were recruited. All data met all assumptions for normality, homoscedasticity, and outlier assumptions. Sex specific demographic and anthropometric characteristics are listed in Table 2.

Table 2. Demographic and anthropometric characteristics.

Variables	All Participants ($n = 46$) Mean ± SD [range]
Age (years)	14.56 ± 1.69; [12.00–18.00]
Height (cm)	165.65 ± 10.05; [147.00–188.00]
Weight (kg)	60.44 ± 13.57; [38.20, 93.80]
BMI (kg/m^2)	21.88 ± 3.91; [16.20–33.40]
BMI Percentiles (%)	61.89 ± 26.35; [9.00, 98.00]
Bodyfat % (DXA)	24.27 ±8.35; [13.20, 45.10]
Pubertal Level (PDS)	2.71 ± 0.81; [0.00, 4.00]
K4b^2 VO$_{2max}$ (mL/kg/min)	42.29 ± 8.37; [20.99, 54.09]
PACER VO$_{2max}$ Estimate (mL/kg/min)	42.67 ± 7.49; [25.88, 54.20]
NET VO$_{2max}$ Estimate (mL/kg/min)	49.82 ± 7.67; [33.11, 60.99]

Pearson correlation coefficients as well as ICC and SEE values are listed in Table 3. Scatterplots depicting the correlations are listed in Figure 1. All assessment methods demonstrated moderate to strong statistically significant correlations and levels of agreement as defined by Portney and Watkins [27] for correlations and Koo and Lee [28] for ICC.

Table 3. Correlation matrix between oxygen consumption estimates per test for both sexes combined.

	Correlations		
	PACER	NET	K4B^2
PACER			
NET	$r = 0.81; p < 0.001$ $r^2 = 0.65$ ICC = 0.72 SEE = 8.53 mL/kg/min [0.57, 0.99]		
K4B^2	$r = 0.87; p < 0.001$ $r^2 = 0.75$ ICC = 0.93 SEE = 4.17 mL/kg/min [0.70, 1.0]	$r = 0.73; p < 0.001$ $r^2 = 0.53$ ICC = 0.67 SEE = 9.56 mL/kg/min [0.50, 0.97]	

A

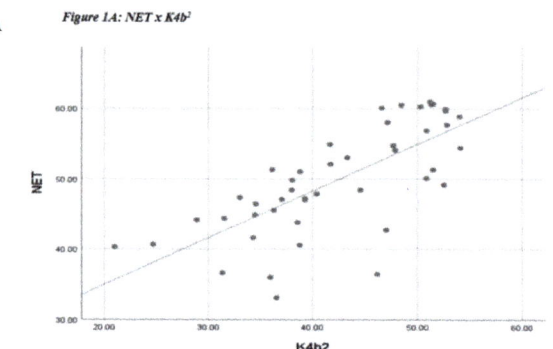

Figure 1A: NET x K4b^2

Figure 1. Cont.

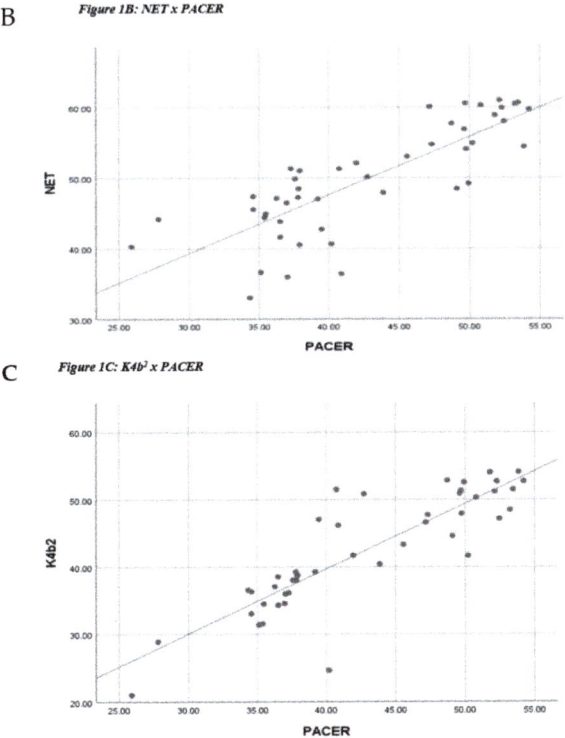

Figure 1. Simple scatterplots. (**A**) NET & K4b^2: $r = 0.73$; (**B**) NET & PACER®: $r = 0.81$; (**C**) K4b^2 & PACER®: $r = 0.87$; Bland–Altman plots (Figure 2) and paired sample t-tests demonstrated acceptable limits of agreement and no significant difference for K4b$^{2\text{TM}}$ and PACER® measures of VO$_{2\text{max}}$ (Figure 2A) (mean difference = -0.37, $t(45) = -0.61$, $p = 0.55$) but showed that the NET VO$_{2\text{max}}$ estimates tend to be overestimated, seen by the upward shift of the mean difference line away from zero, and significantly different in the NET − PACER® (Figure 2B) (mean difference = 7.14, $t(45) = 10.26$, $p < 0.001$) and the NET − K4b$^{2\text{TM}}$ (Figure 2C) (mean difference = 7.52, $t(45) = 8.54$, $p < 0.001$) plots.

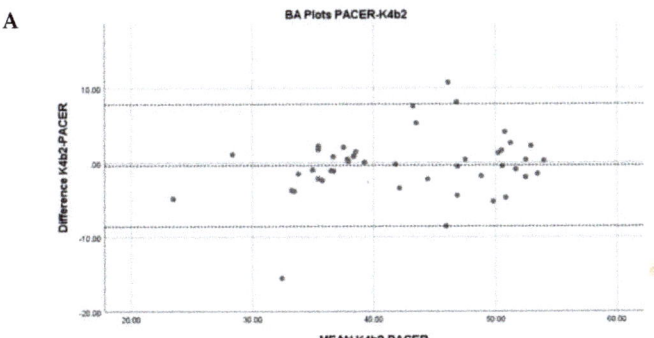

Figure 2. *Cont.*

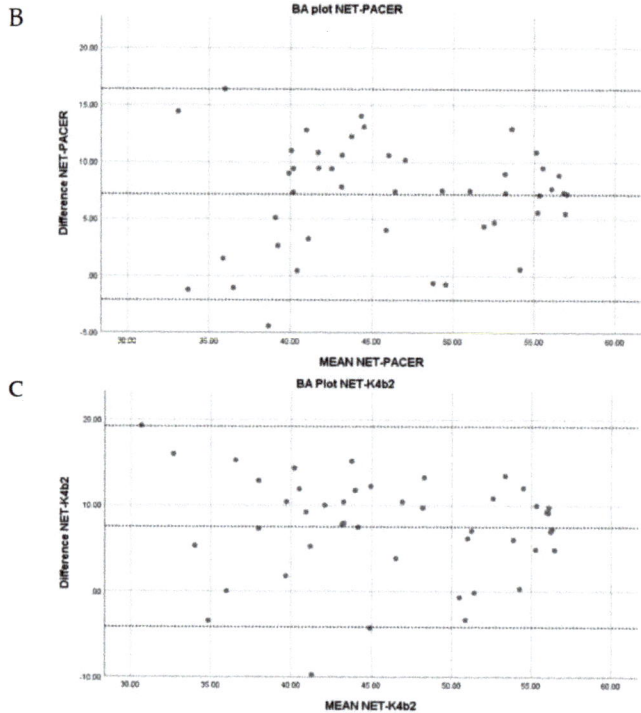

Figure 2. Bland–Altman plots. Middle line represents mean difference while other dotted lines represent the limits of agreement: ±1.96s. (**A**) K4b^2 & PACER®: mean difference = −0.37, limits of agreement of −8.61 & 7.85; (**B**) NET & PACER®: mean difference = 7.14, limits of agreement of −2.10 & 16.39; (**C**) K4b^2 & NET: mean difference = 7.52, limits of agreement of −4.19 & 19.23.

4. Discussion

The aim of this study was to estimate the concurrent validity of the NET for adolescents against the PACER® and objective measures of VO_{2max} as well as to examine the concurrent validity of the VO_{2max} estimation by the PACER® with the VO_{2max} from the K4b$^{2\text{TM}}$ portable metabolic system during the PACER® test. Past studies have shown that the NET is a valid measure of CRF in adult populations [21,22], and our results show that the NET is a valid predictor of VO_{2max} in the adolescent population. This is important, as it offers a quick, easy, inexpensive, and risk-free method of assessing CRF in adolescents. To our knowledge, this is the first report to measure CRF in adolescents without requiring any form of exertion from the participant, which allows for widespread use among large groups and offers a feasible tool for CRF measurement in healthcare settings.

The PACER® test has been validated several times [16,19,20], and our results comparing it to the direct measure of VO_{2max} from the K4b$^{2\text{TM}}$ (r = 0.87) align with past results (r = 0.62–0.83) acquired directly from treadmill maximal exercise tests [16,19,20]. Our study offers a different perspective, as most studies compare the PACER® estimate to a traditional treadmill maximal exercise test, but our research compared the estimate to the direct measure of VO_{2max} acquired at the same time the participant was performing the PACER®. This further strengthens the validity of the PACER® as an indirect measure of VO_{2max} and shows that the PACER® protocol is a valid substitute for a maximally graded exercise test.

In practice, the NET could offer schools a quick and inexpensive tool to assess CRF more frequently than the PACER® test allows, providing valuable information to implement changes in physical education. At the clinical level, the NET can be implemented into healthcare settings as a snapshot of current CRF and can be used as a tool to assess risk for cardiovascular and cardiometabolic disease [1–5].

For efficient use in either setting, the NET results can be analyzed similar to the PACER®, which groups students based on having sufficient or insufficient CRF into the healthy fitness zone (HFZ), the needs improvement zone (NIZ), or the health risk zone (HRZ) [18]. Based on our results, the group values for the zones could be adjusted with the linear regression equation: PACER® = 10.92 + 0.96(NET). For example, a 10-year-old male with a NET score of 46.82–49.42 would fall into the NIZ, a score of ≤46.81 would put him in the HRZ, and a score ≥49.43 would place him into the HFZ. This would allow for a quick assessment to deduce whether an adolescent patient is at risk and requires intervention.

As seen with the Bland–Altman plots and t-tests, the NET VO_{2max} estimates were generally much higher and were significantly different than the values acquired directly through the K4b^{2TM} or estimated through the PACER®. This could be due to the fact the descriptions of the physical activity levels were intended for adults, so it may not have been directly relatable to adolescents. Also, the added weight of the K4b^{2TM} unit, weighing roughly 1 kg, plus the addition of the mask could have resulted in a decreased outcome during the PACER® test. While the NET measures of VO_{2max} were significantly higher, the moderately strong levels of agreement show that the NET is valid and by using the CRF grouping suggested above, as is used by the PACER®, the NET overestimation is inconsequential.

Limitations of this study include a small sample of females and males, thus limiting the ability to fully explore sexes separately, and the running of the PACER® test individually instead of in groups, as is the norm in schools, thus potentially affecting participants' motivation to maximally exert themselves. Regardless of the limitations of this study, there are several strengths in our design and findings, including validating the NET against two different validated measures of VO_{2max} and testing a representative sample of adolescents. Future studies on using the NET for adolescents could examine a larger sample size, perhaps in public schools, to compare against the PACER® or investigate the NET's sensitivity to change in an adolescent's CRF. Future studies need to also assess the reliability of the NET in adolescents, so it can be established as a tool to measure CRF over time.

5. Conclusions

This article gives researchers, clinicians, and coaches a simple, quick, and inexpensive tool to indirectly estimate VO_{2max} in the adolescent population as opposed to a time-consuming and exhausting exercise test. This article also strengthens the evidence for use of the PACER® test as an indirect measure of VO_{2max}, as it provided ventilatory gas analysis during the test itself, showing that the PACER® is a valid graded maximal exertion exercise test, as direct measures of VO_{2max} acquired during performing the PACER® were in agreement with PACER® estimates based on regression equations established against the more traditional treadmill VO_{2max} tests.

Author Contributions: Conceptualization: A.O., L.K., P.M.; Methodology: A.O.; Formal Analysis: P.M.; Investigation: P.M., M.C., A.B., A.F. L.K., A.O., W.B.; Resources: L.K., A.O., W.B.; Data Curation: P.M., M.C.; Writing—Original Draft Preparation: P.M.; Writing—Review and Editing: P.M., A.O., L.K.; Supervision: A.O., L.K., W.B.

Funding: This study was funded by the Texas Physical Therapy Foundation. The results of this study are presented clearly, honestly, and without fabrication, falsification, or inappropriate data manipulation. The results from this study do not constitute endorsement by the Texas Physical Therapy Association.

Conflicts of Interest: The authors have no conflict of interest to disclose.

References

1. Parrett, A.L.; Valentine, R.J.; Arngrimsson, S.A.; Castelli, D.M.; Evans, E.M. Adiposity and aerobic fitness are associated with metabolic disease risk in children. *Appl. Physiol. Nutr. Metab.* **2011**, *36*, 72–79. [CrossRef] [PubMed]
2. Lukacs, A.; Varga, B.; Kiss-Toth, E.; Soos, A.; Barkai, L. Factors influencing the diabetes-specific health-related quality of life in children and adolescents with type 1 diabetes mellitus. *J. Child Heal. Care* **2014**, *18*, 253–260. [CrossRef] [PubMed]

3. Twisk, J.W.R.; Kemper, H.C.G.; Mechelen, W. Van Tracking of activity and fitness and the relationship with cardiovascular disease risk factors. *Med. Sci. Sport. Exerc.* **2000**, 1455–1461. [CrossRef]
4. Houston, E.L.; Baker, J.S.; Buchan, D.S.; Stratton, G.; Fairclough, S.J.; Foweather, L.; Gobbi, R.; Graves, L.E.F.; Hopkins, N.; Boddy, L.M. Cardiorespiratory fitness predicts clustered cardiometabolic risk in 10–11.9-year-olds. *Eur. J. Pediatr.* **2013**, *172*, 913–918. [CrossRef] [PubMed]
5. Bailey, D.P.; Boddy, L.M.; Savory, L.A.; Denton, S.J.; Kerr, C.J. Associations between cardiorespiratory fitness, physical activity and clustered cardiometabolic risk in children and adolescents: The HAPPY study. *Eur. J. Pediatr.* **2012**, *171*, 1317–1323. [CrossRef] [PubMed]
6. Chaddock, L.; Hillman, C.H.; Pontifex, M.B.; Johnson, C.R.; Raine, L.B.; Kramer, A.F. Childhood aerobic fitness predicts cognitive performance one year later. *J. Sports Sci.* **2012**, *30*, 421–430. [CrossRef] [PubMed]
7. Haapala, E.A. Cardiorespiratory Fitness and Motor Skills in Relation to Cognition and Academic Performance in Children – A Review by. *J. Hum. Kinet.* **2013**, *36*, 55–68. [CrossRef]
8. Chaddock, L.; Erickson, K.I.; Prakash, R.S.; Vanpatter, M.; Voss, M.W.; Pontifex, M.B.; Raine, L.B.; Hillman, C.H.; Kramer, A.F. Basal ganglia volume is associated with aerobic fitness in preadolescent children. *Dev. Neurosci.* **2010**, *32*, 249–256. [CrossRef]
9. Hillman, C.H.; Erickson, K.I.; Kramer, A.F. Be smart, exercise your heart: exercise effects on brain and cognition. *Nat. Rev. Neurosci.* **2008**, *9*, 58–65. [CrossRef]
10. Pontifex, M.B.; Raine, L.B.; Johnson, C.R.; Chaddock, L.; Voss, M.W.; Cohen, N.; Kramer, A.F.; Hillman, C.H. Cardiorespiratory Fitness and the Flexible Modulation of Cognitive Control in Preadolescent Children. *J. Cogn. Neurosci.* **2010**, *23*, 1332–1345. [CrossRef]
11. Chaddock, L.; Erickson, K.I.; Prakash, R.S.; Kim, J.S.; Voss, M.W.; VanPatter, M.; Pontifex, M.B.; Raine, L.B.; Konkel, A.; Hillman, C.H.; et al. A neuroimaging investigation of the association between aerobic fitness, hippocampal volume, and memory performance in preadolescent children. *Brain Res.* **2014**, *1358*, 172–183. [CrossRef] [PubMed]
12. Huotari, P.; Nupponen, H.; Mikkelsson, L.; Laakso, L.; Kujala, U. Adolescent physical fitness and activity as predictors of adulthood activity. *J. Sports Sci.* **2011**, *29*, 1135–1141. [CrossRef] [PubMed]
13. Jose, K.A.; Blizzard, L.; Dwyer, T.; Mckercher, C.; Venn, A.J. Childhood and adolescent predictors of leisure time physical activity during the transition from adolescence to adulthood: A population based cohort study. *Int. J. Behav. Nutr. Phys. Act.* **2011**, *8*, 1–9. [CrossRef] [PubMed]
14. Davis, J. Direct determination of aerobic power. In *Physiological Assessment of Human Fitness*; Human Kinetics: Champaign, IL, USA, 1995; pp. 9–17.
15. Ward, A.; Ebbeling, C.; Ahlquist, L. Indirect methods for estimation of aerobic power. In *Physiological Assessment of Human Fitness*; Human Kinetics: Champaign, IL, USA, 1995; pp. 37–56.
16. Van Mechelen, W.; Hlobil, H.; Kemper, H.C.G. Validation of two running tests as estimates of maximal aerobic power in children. *Eur. J. Appl. Physiol.* **1986**, *55*, 503–506. [CrossRef]
17. Mayorga-Vega, D.; Aguilar-Soto, P.; Viciana, J. Criterion-related validity of the 20-m shuttle run test for estimating cardiorespiratory fitness: A meta-analysis. *J. Sport. Sci. Med.* **2015**, *14*, 536–547.
18. Meredith, M.; Welk, G. *FITNESSGRAM®/ACTIVITYGRAM® Test Administration Manual*, 4th ed.; Human Kinetics: Champaign, IL, USA, 2013; Available online: www.cooperinstitute.org/vault/2440/web/files/662.pdf (accessed on 31 December 2017).
19. Kabiri, L.S.; Mitchell, K.; Brewer, W.; Ortiz, A. Muscular and Cardiorespiratory Fitness in Homeschool versus Public School Children Running. *Pediatr. Exerc. Sci.* **2017**, *29*, 371–376. [CrossRef] [PubMed]
20. Mahar, M.T.; Welk, G.J.; Rowe, D.A.; Crotts, D.J.; Mciver, K.L. Development and Validation of a Regres- sion Model to Estimate VO_2peak From PACER 20-m Shuttle Run Performance. *J. Phys. Act. Health* **2006**, *3*, 34–46. [CrossRef]
21. Jurca, R.; Jackson, A.S.; Lamonte, M.J.; Morrow, J.R., Jr.; Blair, S.N.; Wareham, N.J.; Haskell, W.L.; Van Mechelen, W.; Church, T.S.; Jakicic, J.M. Assessing Cardiorespiratory Fitness Without Performing Exercise Testing. *Am. J. Prev. Med.* **2005**, *29*, 185–193. [CrossRef]
22. Jackson, A.S.; Sui, X.; Connor, D.P.O.; Church, T.S.; Lee, D.; Artero, E.G.; Blair, S.N. Longitudinal Cardiorespiratory Fitness Alogrithms for Clinical Settings. *Am. J. Prev. Med.* **2012**, *43*, 512–519. [CrossRef]
23. Duffield, R.; Dawson, B.; Pinnington, H.; Wong, P. Accuracy and reliabillity of a Cosmed K4b 2 portable gas aScience, Exercisenalysis system. *J. Sci. Med. Sport* **2004**, *7*, 11–22. [CrossRef]

24. Schrack, J.A.; Simonsick, E.M.; Ferrucci, L. Comparison of the Cosmed K4b2 Portable Metabolic System in Measuring Steady-State Walking Energy Expenditure. *PLoS ONE* **2010**, *5*, 2–6. [CrossRef] [PubMed]
25. Silva, G.; Oliveira, N.L.; Aires, L.; Mota, J.; Oliveira, J.; Ribeiro, J.C. Calculation and validation of models for estimating VO_{2max} from the 20-m shuttle run test in children and adolescents Gustavo. *Arch. Exerc. Heal. Dis.* **2012**, *2*, 145–152. [CrossRef]
26. Mahar, M.T.; Guerieri, A.M.; Hanna, M.S.; Kemble, C.D. Estimation of Aerobic Fitness from 20-m Multistage Shuttle Run Test Performance. *Am. J. Prev. Med.* **2011**, *41*, S117–S123. [CrossRef] [PubMed]
27. Portney, L.G.; Watkins, M.P. *Foundations of Clinical Research: Applications to Practice*, 3rd ed.; F.A. Davis Company: Philadelphia, PA, USA, 2015; p. 525.
28. Koo, T.K.; Li, M.Y. A Guideline of Selecting and Reporting Intraclass Correlation Coefficients for Reliability Research. *J. Chiropr. Med.* **2016**, *15*, 155–163. [CrossRef] [PubMed]

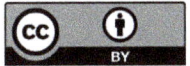

© 2019 by the authors. Licensee MDPI, Basel, Switzerland. This article is an open access article distributed under the terms and conditions of the Creative Commons Attribution (CC BY) license (http://creativecommons.org/licenses/by/4.0/).

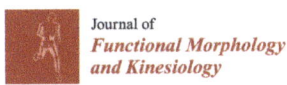

Article

Anthropometric Obesity Indices, Body Fat Percentage, and Grip Strength in Young Adults with different Physical Activity Levels

Mustafa Söğüt [1], Ömer Barış Kaya [1], Kübra Altunsoy [1], Cain C. T. Clark [2,*], Filipe Manuel Clemente [3,4] and Ali Ahmet Doğan [1]

1. Faculty of Sport Sciences, Kırıkkale University, Kırıkkale 71450 Turkey
2. Centre for Sport, Exercise and Life Sciences, Coventry University, Coventry CV1 5FB, UK
3. Polytechnic Institute of Viana do Castelo, School of Sport and Leisure, 4960-320 Melgaço, Portugal
4. Instituto de Telecomunicações, 6200-001 Delegação da Covilhã, Portugal
* Correspondence: cain.clark@coventry.ac.uk

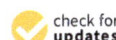

Received: 5 July 2019; Accepted: 30 July 2019; Published: 31 July 2019

Abstract: The purposes of this study were to determine whether moderately physically active (MPA) and highly physically active (HPA) male (n = 96, age = 22.5 ± 1.7 years) and female (n = 85, age = 21.3 ± 1.6 years) young adults differed in their anthropometric obesity indices (AOIs), body fat percentage (BF%), and muscular strength, and also to examine the associations between physical activity level (PAL) and the abovementioned variables. Participants were measured for body height and weight, BF%, waist and hip circumferences, and maximal isometric grip strength. According to their PAL, estimated by the short version of the International Physical Activity Questionnaire, they were assigned to MPA and HPA subgroups. Regardless of gender, results indicated that participants in the MPA groups had significantly higher values of body weight, waist and hip circumference, BF%, and BMI than participants in the HPA groups. No significant differences were found between physical activity groups in terms of grip strength. The AOIs and BF% were found to be significantly and negatively correlated with the PAL in both genders. In conclusion, the findings of the study suggest that high habitual physical activity is associated with lower adiposity markers. However, the differences in the hand grip strength of the contrasting activity groups were negligible.

Keywords: obesity indices; body composition; grip strength; physical activity

1. Introduction

The consequences of physical inactivity, including a diverse range of chronic and non-communicable diseases is well-documented, such as coronary heart disease [1], breast and colon cancers [2,3], osteoporosis [4], noninsulin-dependent diabetes [5], excess adiposity [6], depression [7], and all-cause mortality [8]. Nevertheless, sedentary lifestyle behaviors are still common worldwide [9], and it presents a major global public health concern.

Accumulating evidence suggests that habitual physical activity has a positive influence on various health outcomes [10–12]. The findings of large, recent cohort studies have indicated that physical activity level (PAL) is inversely associated with body fat percentage (BF%), body mass index (BMI), and/or other adiposity indicators [13–16]. Notwithstanding, inconsistent results have been observed in certain age groups with regard to the relationship between physical activity and muscular strength [17–20].

Muscular strength is a determinant of physical quality that ensures a lower cardiovascular risk factor [21], a healthy mineral bone density, and high levels of lean mass [22], independently of other fitness variables or sociodemographic measures. Despite there being many ways to assess muscular strength, one of the most common tests carried out in adults is grip strength, which is an important clinical and prognostic value [23]. Usually, strong and positive correlations have been found between hand grip strength and muscle mass [24]. On the other hand, low hand grip strength is associated with increased risk of functional limitations and disability in one's later years, as well as a general cause of mortality [25]. In spite of such evidence, there is a lack of studies testing the relationship between PALs and strength, and this should be considered to understand the mechanism that explains good maintenance of strength.

Although young adulthood is a critical developmental period characterized by important changes in health status, such as unhealthy weight gain [26,27] and physical inactivity [28], the majority of the relevant examinations have been conducted with children and older adults. Thus, current literature provides limited evidence on the disparities in adiposity and muscular strength in university students with different PALs. Therefore, the purposes of the present study were to examine whether moderately physically active (MPA) and highly physically active (HPA) male and female young adults differed in their anthropometric obesity indices (AOIs), BF%, and muscular strength, and to analyze the relations between PAL and the aforementioned variables.

2. Materials and Methods

2.1. Participants

A cohort of male (n = 96, age = 22.5 ± 1.7 years) and female (n = 85, age = 21.3 ± 1.6 years) university students from a state university located in central Anatolia (Turkey) were recruited to take part in the study. They were initially briefed of the measurement procedures and the aims of the study, and then requested to sign informed consent forms. Ethical approval was obtained from the Non-interventional Researches Ethics Board of Kırıkkale University (approval number/identification code of the study is 2019.06.25).

2.2. Anthropometric Measurements

Anthropometric assessments were performed in accordance with standardized procedures [29]. Body height was measured with a portable stadiometer (Seca 213, Hamburg, Germany) to the nearest 0.1 cm. Body mass (0.1 kg) and BF% were evaluated by a bioelectrical impedance analyzer (Tanita, BC-418, Japan). Waist and hip circumferences were measured with a flexible steel tape to the nearest centimeter at the smallest circumference between the ribs and the iliac crest and at the level of maximum protuberance of the buttocks, respectively. BMI was calculated by dividing the body weight (kg) by the body height squared (m).

2.3. Grip Strength

A digital hand dynamometer (T.K.K.5401 Grip-D, Takei, Japan) was used to assess maximal isometric grip strength. Participants were asked to stay in a standing position and keep one arm straight and parallel to the body. They were requested to hold the dynamometer with their dominant hand and squeeze the handle as hard as possible for three seconds. The highest value acquired from the three trials was used for the analysis.

2.4. Physical Activity

The PAL of the participants was estimated via the short form of the International Physical Activity Questionnaire (IPAQ) [30,31]. The IPAQ requires respondents to recall the frequency, duration, and intensity of physical activity they engaged in during the last seven days. Each type of activity (moderate- and vigorous-intensity walking) was then converted to metabolic equivalent (MET) minutes, enabling the determination of total weekly physical activity. Based on their weekly MET minutes, they were divided into two groups—MPA (≥600–3000 MET min/week) and HPA (≥3000 MET min/week) [30,31].

2.5. Statistical Analysis

Data were analyzed using SPSS for Windows. Descriptive statistics (mean ± SD) were calculated for all variables. An independent sample t-test was used to ascertain differences between PAL groups. Effect sizes (ES) were quantified to determine the magnitude of differences. Based on the Cohen's d values, ES were considered as: <0.20 (trivial), 0.20 to 0.59 (small), 0.60 to 1.19 (moderate), 1.20 to 1.99 (large), 2.0 to 3.9 (very large), and >4.0 (extremely large) [32]. A Pearson correlation coefficient was conducted to examine the associations between PAL and other variables. Correlations were categorized as 0.0–0.1 (trivial), 0.1–0.3 (small), 0.3–0.5 (moderate), 0.5–0.7 (large), 0.7–0.9 (very large), and 0.9–1.0 (near perfect) [32].

3. Results

Descriptive statistics (mean ± SD), t-test results, and effect sizes for male and female participants are presented in Tables 1 and 2. Results highlighted that participants in the HPA groups had significantly lower values in BF%, body mass, waist and hip circumference, and BMI than the participants in the MPA groups in both genders. There were no significant differences in age, body height, and grip strength results between groups.

Table 1. Descriptive statistics, t-test results, and effect size values for male participants.

Physical Activity Groups	MPA (n = 45)	HPA (n = 51)	t	p	d
Age (years)	22.8 (1.8)	22.2 (1.6)	1.861	0.066	0.38
Activity (MET m/w)	1922.1 (799.2)	4883.1 (1203.3)	−14.001	0.001	−2.89
Height (cm)	175.2 (6.3)	175.1 (6.8)	0.082	0.935	0.02
Weight (kg)	71.9 (8.1)	68.4 (7.5)	2.245	0.027	0.46
Waist (cm)	80.1 (5.7)	77.1 (4.9)	2.707	0.008	0.55
Hip (cm)	96.2 (4.8)	93.7 (5.4)	2.347	0.021	0.46
BMI (kg/m^2)	23.50 (2.7)	22.34 (2.2)	2.285	0.025	0.46
Body fat (%)	13.5 (5.8)	10.5 (3.8)	3.275	0.001	0.67
Grip strength (kg)	47.5 (7.0)	47.9 (6.8)	−0.291	0.772	−0.06

Table 2. Descriptive statistics, t-test results, and effect size values for female participants.

Physical Activity Groups	MPA (n = 37)	HPA (n = 48)	t	p	d
Age (years)	21.2 (1.7)	21.3 (1.6)	−0.324	0.747	−0.07
Activity (MET m/w)	1665.3 (777.5)	4863.2 (821.2)	−18.214	0.001	−3.98
Height (cm)	162.1 (5.6)	161.2 (6.6)	0.705	0.483	0.15
Weight (kg)	60.8 (11.9)	54.8 (8.7)	2.646	0.010	0.58
Waist (cm)	69.9 (8.1)	66.7 (5.2)	2.184	0.032	0.48
Hip (cm)	96.8 (7.8)	93.3 (6.3)	2.257	0.027	0.49
BMI (kg/m^2)	23.05 (4.2)	21.03 (2.7)	2.703	0.008	0.59
Body fat (%)	27.6 (8.1)	22.4 (6.5)	3.301	0.001	0.72
Grip strength (kg)	27.2 (4.4)	27.3 (3.8)	−0.182	0.856	−0.04

Table 3 presents the correlation coefficients between PAL and other variables for each gender, separately. Results indicated that the PAL, regardless of gender, was found to be significantly and negatively correlated with all AOIs and BF%. On the other hand, no significant associations were found between PAL and grip strength values in both male and female participants.

Table 3. Correlation results between physical activity level (PAL) and other variables by gender.

Variables	Male		Female	
	r	p	r	p
Height	0.012	0.905	−0.016	0.886
Weight	−0.211	0.039	−0.304	0.005
Waist	−0.373	0.001	−0.246	0.023
Hip	−0.284	0.005	−0.296	0.006
BMI	−0.227	0.026	−0.342	0.001
BF%	−0.432	0.001	−0.398	0.001
Grip strength	−0.033	0.746	0.100	0.364

4. Discussion

The aim of the present study was to investigate the possible differences in various adiposity parameters and muscular strength in a group of young male and female adults with distinct physical activity profiles. The results of the study indicated that the participants in the HPA group had significantly lower values in all AOIs and BF% than their MPA counterparts in both genders. Furthermore, regardless of gender, PAL was found to be significantly and negatively correlated with AOIs and BF%. The results, with regard to reported correlation coefficients, are in line with the findings of previous longitudinal [33–35] and cross-sectional [36,37] examinations. Concordant with our findings, results of some recent work noted similar observations, that individuals who engaged in greater physical activity were found to have preferential indices of adiposity [13,14].

The results demonstrated that there were no significant differences in grip strength results between activity groups. This observation is in accord with the findings of previous studies conducted with children [38], young adults [39], and older adults [40]. Furthermore, no significant associations were obtained between PAL and grip strength values in both genders. This might conceivably be attributed to comparable body sizes, where trivial and small magnitudes of differences were found between groups for body height and weight, respectively. Furthermore, the participants were grouped by the IPAQ, which does not specifically assess participation in strengthening activities, so may not be sufficiently sensitive. In addition, other possible anthropometric correlates of hand grip strength that were not measured in this study, such as hand size and forearm circumference [41], total arm length and upper arm circumference [42], and hand circumference [43] might contribute to this insignificance, and therefore warrants further examination.

With regard to practical implications, it is conceivable that high PALs and good levels of strength may help to maintain health levels across adulthood. Different studies have suggested that upper and lower body muscular strength are important factors that contribute to a lower risk of mortality in the adult population, regardless of age [44,45]. Although no differences were found between PALs in strength, it is important to highlight that strength is an independent physical quality and should be worked out concurrently with other fitness components (e.g., cardiorespiratory fitness). Thus, a healthy lifestyle should include both cardiorespiratory and muscular strength training/stimuli [46].

5. Conclusions

The findings of the present study revealed that higher levels of habitual physical activity is associated with lower adiposity markers in young adults. Nevertheless, differences in hand grip strength of the contrasting activity groups were negligible. It should also be acknowledged that the current study has several limitations. Firstly, the subjective assessment may cause incorrect estimation of physical activity; however, use of the well-validated IPAQ ameliorates some concern. Secondly, in spite of its important advantages (i.e., being relatively inexpensive, portable, and quick), rather than BIA, criterion methods such as underwater weighing or dual-energy x-ray absorptiometry might be used to determine body fat, but nevertheless present significant time and cost restrictions. Nevertheless, it is recommended that future studies expand this observation through using a larger sample and more complex reference methods to measure physical activity levels and body composition.

Author Contributions: Conceptualization, M.S. and O.B.K.; Data curation, M.S. and O.B.K.; Formal analysis, M.S.; Investigation, K.A. and F.M.C.; Software, M.S.; Supervision, C.C.T.C. and A.A.D.; Writing—original draft, M.S., O.B.K., K.A., C.C.T.C. and F.M.C.; Writing—review and editing, C.C.T.C. and A.A.D.

Funding: This research received no external funding.

Conflicts of Interest: The authors declare no conflict of interest.

References

1. Sattelmair, J.; Pertman, J.; Ding, E.L.; Kohl, H.W., III; Haskell, W.; Lee, I.M. Dose response between physical activity and risk of coronary heart disease: A meta-analysis. *Circulation* **2011**, *124*, 789–795. [CrossRef] [PubMed]
2. Friedenreich, C.M. Physical activity and breast cancer: Review of the epidemiologic evidence and biologic mechanisms. *Recent Results Cancer Res.* **2011**, *188*, 125–139. [PubMed]
3. Wolin, K.Y.; Yan, Y.; Colditz, G.A.; Lee, I.M. Physical activity and colon cancer prevention: A meta-analysis. *Br. J. Cancer* **2009**, *100*, 611. [CrossRef] [PubMed]
4. Lane, N.E. Epidemiology, etiology, and diagnosis of osteoporosis. *Am. J. Obstet. Gynecol.* **2006**, *19*, S3–S11. [CrossRef] [PubMed]
5. Jeon, C.Y.; Lokken, R.P.; Hu, F.B.; Van Dam, R.M. Physical activity of moderate intensity and risk of type 2 diabetes: A systematic review. *Diabetes Care* **2007**, *30*, 744–752. [PubMed]
6. Pietiläinen, K.H.; Kaprio, J.; Borg, P.; Plasqui, G.; Yki-Järvinen, H.; Kujala, U.M.; Rose, R.J.; Westerterp, K.R.; Rissanen, A. Physical inactivity and obesity: A vicious circle. *Obesity* **2008**, *16*, 409–414. [CrossRef] [PubMed]
7. Weyerer, S. Physical Inactivity and Depression in the Community. *Int. J. Sports Med.* **1992**, *13*, 492–496. [CrossRef]
8. Lollgen, H.; Bockenhoff, A.; Knapp, G. Physical activity and all-cause mortality: An updated metaanalysis with different intensity categories. *Int. J. Sports Med.* **2009**, *30*, 213–224. [CrossRef]
9. Hallal, P.C.; Andersen, L.B.; Bull, F.C.; Guthold, R.; Haskell, W.; Ekelund, U.; Lancet Physical Activity Series Working Group. Global physical activity levels: Surveillance progress, pitfalls, and prospects. *Lancet* **2012**, *380*, 247–257. [CrossRef]
10. Blair, S.N.; Cheng, Y.; Holder, J.S. Is physical activity or physical fitness more important in defining health benefits? *Med. Sci. Sports Exerc.* **2001**, *33*, 379–399.
11. Reiner, M.; Niermann, C.; Jekauc, D.; Woll, A. Long-term health benefits of physical activity—A systematic review of longitudinal studies. *BMC Public Health* **2013**, *13*, 813. [CrossRef]
12. Warburton, D.E.; Nicol, C.W.; Bredin, S.S. Health benefits of physical activity: The evidence. *Can. Med. Assoc. J.* **2006**, *174*, 801–809. [CrossRef] [PubMed]
13. Besson, H.; Ekelund, U.; Luan, J.; May, A.M.; Sharp, S.; Travier, N.; Agudo, A.; Slimani, N.; Rinaldi, S.; Jenab, M.; et al. A cross-sectional analysis of physical activity and obesity indicators in European participants of the EPIC-PANACEA study. *Int. J. Obes.* **2009**, *33*, 497–506. [CrossRef] [PubMed]
14. Maher, C.A.; Mire, E.; Harrington, D.M.; Staiano, A.E.; Katzmarzyk, P.T. The independent and combined associations of physical activity and sedentary behavior with obesity in adults: NHANES 2003-06. *Obesity* **2013**, *21*, 730–737. [CrossRef] [PubMed]
15. Moliner-Urdiales, D.; Ruiz, J.R.; Ortega, F.B.; Rey-Lopez, J.P.; Vicente-Rodríguez, G.; España-Romero, V.; Izquierdo, D.M.; Castillo, M.J.; Sjöström, M.; Moreno, L.A. Association of objectively assessed physical activity with total and central body fat in Spanish adolescents; The HELENA Study. *Int. J. Obes.* **2009**, *33*, 1126–1135. [CrossRef]
16. Ruiz, J.R.; Rizzo, N.S.; Hurtig-Wennlöf, A.; Ortega, F.B.; Wàrnberg, J.; Sjöström, M. Relations of total physical activity and intensity to fitness and fatness in children: The European Youth Heart Study. *Am. J. Clin. Nutr.* **2006**, *84*, 299–303. [CrossRef]

17. Bann, D.; Hire, D.; Manini, T.; Cooper, R.; Botoseneanu, A.; McDermott, M.M.; Pahor, M.; Glynn, N.W.; Fielding, R.; King, A.C.; et al. Light intensity physical activity and sedentary behavior in relation to body mass index and grip strength in older adults: Cross-sectional findings from the lifestyle interventions and independence for elders (LIFE) study. *PLoS ONE* **2015**, *10*, e0116058.
18. Cooper, A.J.M.; Lamb, M.J.E.; Sharp, S.J.; Simmons, R.K.; Griffin, S.J. Bidirectional association between physical activity and muscular strength in older adults: Results from the UK Biobank study. *Int. J. Epidemiol.* **2016**, *46*, 141–148.
19. Martin, H.J.; Syddall, H.E.; Dennison, E.M.; Cooper, C.; Sayer, A.A. Relationship between customary physical activity, muscle strength and physical performance in older men and women: Findings from the Hertfordshire Cohort Study. *Age Ageing* **2008**, *37*, 589–593. [CrossRef]
20. Westbury, L.D.; Dodds, R.M.; Syddall, H.E.; Baczynska, A.M.; Shaw, S.C.; Dennison, E.M.; Roberts, H.C.; Sayer, A.A.; Cooper, C.; Patel, H.P. Associations Between Objectively Measured Physical Activity, Body Composition and Sarcopenia: Findings from the Hertfordshire Sarcopenia Study (HSS). *Calcif. Tissue Int.* **2018**, *103*, 237–245.
21. Grøntved, A.; Ried-Larsen, M.; Møller, N.C.; Kristensen, P.L.; Froberg, K.; Brage, S.; Andersen, L.B. Muscle strength in youth and cardiovascular risk in young adulthood (the European Youth Heart Study). *Br. J. Sports Med.* **2015**, *49*, 90–94. [CrossRef]
22. Guimarães, B.R.; Pimenta, L.D.; Massini, D.A.; Dos Santos, D.; da Cruz Siqueira, L.O.; Simionato, A.R.; dos Santos, L.G.A.; Neiva, C.M.; Filho, D.M.P. Muscle strength and regional lean body mass influence on mineral bone health in young male adults. *PLoS ONE* **2018**, *13*, e0191769. [CrossRef]
23. Bohannon, R.W. Muscle strength: Clinical and prognostic value of hand-grip dynamometry. *Curr. Opin. Clin. Nutr. Metab. Care* **2015**, *18*, 465–470. [CrossRef]
24. Steffl, M.; Bohannon, R.W.; Houdova, V.; Musalek, M.; Prajerova, K.; Cesak, P.; Petra, M.; Kohlikovaa, E.; Holmerova, I. Association between clinical measures of sarcopenia in a sample of community-dwelling women. *Isokinet. Exerc. Sci.* **2015**, *23*, 41–44. [CrossRef]
25. Norman, K.; Stobäus, N.; Gonzalez, M.C.; Schulzke, J.D.; Pirlich, M. Hand grip strength: Outcome predictor and marker of nutritional status. *Clin. Nutr.* **2011**, *30*, 135–142. [CrossRef]
26. Gordon-Larsen, P.; Adair, L.S.; Nelson, M.C.; Popkin, B.M. Five-year obesity incidence in the transition period between adolescence and adulthood: The National Longitudinal Study of Adolescent Health. *Am. J. Clin. Nutr.* **2004**, *80*, 569–575.
27. Lee, H.; Lee, D.; Guo, G.; Harris, K.M. Trends in body mass index in adolescence and young adulthood in the United States: 1959–2002. *J. Adolesc. Health* **2011**, *49*, 601–608.
28. Telama, R.; Yang, X. Decline of physical activity from youth to young adulthood in Finland. *Med. Sci. Sports Exerc.* **2000**, *32*, 1617–1622. [CrossRef]
29. Lohman, T.G.; Roche, A.F.; Martorell, R. *Anthropometric Standardization Reference Manual*; Human Kinetics: Champaign, IL, USA, 1988.
30. Craig, C.L.; Marshall, A.L.; Sjostrom, M.; Bauman, A.E.; Booth, M.L.; Ainsworth, B.E.; Pratt, M.; Ekelund, U.; Yngve, A.; Sallis, J.F.; et al. International physical activity questionnaire: 12-Country reliability and validity. *Med. Sci. Sports Exer.* **2003**, *35*, 1381–1395. [CrossRef]
31. IPAQ Research Committee. Guidelines for Data Processing and Analysis of the International Physical Activity Questionnaire-Short and Long Forms. 2005. Available online: http://www.ipaq.ki.se (accessed on 5 May 2019).
32. Hopkins, W.G.; Marshall, S.W.; Batterham, A.M.; Hanin, J. Progressive statistics for studies in sports medicine and exercise science. *Med. Sci. Sports Exer.* **2009**, *41*, 3–13. [CrossRef]
33. Bell, A.C.; Ge, K.; Popkin, B.M. Weight gain and its predictors in Chinese adults. *Int. J. Obes.* **2001**, *25*, 1079–1086. [CrossRef]
34. Schmitz, K.H.; Jacobs, D.R., Jr.; Leon, A.S.; Schreiner, P.J.; Sternfeld, B. Physical activity and body weight: Associations over ten years in the CARDIA study. *Int. J. Obes.* **2000**, *24*, 1475–1487. [CrossRef]
35. Wagner, A.; Simon, C.; Ducimetiere, P.; Montaye, M.; Bongard, V.; Yarnell, J.; Bingham, A.; Hedelin, G.; Amouyel, P.; FerrieÁres, J.; et al. Leisure-time physical activity and regular walking or cycling to work are associated with adiposity and 5 y weight gain in middle-aged men: The PRIME Study. *Int. J. Obes.* **2001**, *25*, 940–948. [CrossRef]

36. Bowen, L.; Taylor, A.E.; Sullivan, R.; Ebrahim, S.; Kinra, S.; Krishna, K.R.; Krishna, K.V.R.; Kulkarni, B.; Ben-Shlomo, Y.; Ekelund, U.; et al. Associations between diet, physical activity and body fat distribution: A cross sectional study in an Indian population. *BMC Public Health* **2015**, *15*, 281. [CrossRef]
37. Zanovec, M.; Lakkakula, A.P.; Johnson, L.G.; Turri, G. Physical activity is associated with percent body fat and body composition but not body mass index in white and black college students. *Int. J. Exerc. Sci.* **2009**, *2*, 175–185.
38. Cho, M.; Kim, J.Y. Changes in physical fitness and body composition according to the physical activities of Korean adolescents. *J. Exerc. Rehabil.* **2017**, *13*, 568–572.
39. Mikaelsson, K.; Eliasson, K.; Lysholm, J.; Nyberg, L.; Michaelson, P. Physical capacity in physically active and non-active adolescents. *J. Public Health* **2011**, *19*, 131–138. [CrossRef]
40. Morie, M.; Reid, K.F.; Miciek, R.; Lajevardi, N.; Choong, K.; Krasnoff, J.B.; Storer, T.W.; Fielding, R.A.; Bhasin, S.; Lebrasseur, N.K. Habitual Physical Activity Levels are Associated with Performance in Measures of Physical Function and Mobility in Older Men. *J. Am. Geriatr. Soc.* **2010**, *58*, 1727–1733. [CrossRef]
41. Günther, C.M.; Bürger, A.; Rickert, M.; Crispin, A.; Schulz, C.U. Grip strength in healthy caucasian adults: Reference values. *J. Hand Surg.* **2008**, *33*, 558–565. [CrossRef]
42. Koley, S.; Singh, A.P. An association of dominant hand grip strength with some anthropometric variables in Indian collegiate population. *Anthropol. Anz.* **2009**, *67*, 21–28. [CrossRef]
43. Li, K.; Hewson, D.J.; Duchêne, J.; Hogrel, J.Y. Predicting maximal grip strength using hand circumference. *Man. Ther.* **2010**, *15*, 579–585. [CrossRef]
44. García-Hermoso, A.; Cavero-Redondo, I.; Ramírez-Vélez, R.; Ruiz, J.R.; Ortega, F.B.; Lee, D.C.; Martínez-Vizcaíno, V. Muscular strength as a predictor of all-cause mortality in an apparently healthy population: A systematic review and meta-analysis of data from approximately 2 million men and women. *Arch. Phys. Med. Rehabil.* **2018**, *99*, 2100–2113. [CrossRef]
45. Volaklis, K.A.; Halle, M.; Meisinger, C. Muscular strength as a strong predictor of mortality: A narrative review. *Eur. J. Intern. Med.* **2015**, *26*, 303–310. [CrossRef]
46. Schumann, M.; Yli-Peltola, K.; Abbiss, C.R.; Häkkinen, K. Cardiorespiratory adaptations during concurrent aerobic and strength training in men and women. *PLoS ONE* **2015**, *10*, e0139279. [CrossRef]

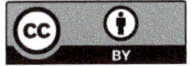

© 2019 by the authors. Licensee MDPI, Basel, Switzerland. This article is an open access article distributed under the terms and conditions of the Creative Commons Attribution (CC BY) license (http://creativecommons.org/licenses/by/4.0/).

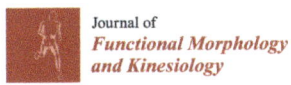

Article

Accelerometer-Based Physical Activity Levels Differ between Week and Weekend Days in British Preschool Children

Clare M. P. Roscoe [1,*], Rob S. James [2] and Michael J. Duncan [2]

1   Human Sciences Research Centre, University of Derby, Kedleston Road, Derby DE22 1GB, UK
2   Centre for Applied Biological and Exercise Sciences, Coventry University, Priory Street, Coventry CV1 5FB, UK; aa8396@coventry.ac.uk (R.S.J.); apx214@coventry.ac.uk (M.J.D.)
*   Correspondence: c.roscoe@derby.ac.uk; Tel.: +44-1332-591284

Received: 10 August 2019; Accepted: 7 September 2019; Published: 12 September 2019

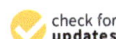

Abstract: Participation in physical activity (PA) is fundamental to children's future health. Studies examining the temporal pattern of PA between weekdays and weekends in British preschool children are lacking. Therefore, the aim of this study was to compare PA levels between week and weekend days for UK preschool children, using objective measurements. One hundred and eighty-five preschool children (99 boys, 86 girls, aged 4–5 years), from central England wore a triaxial accelerometer (GENEActiv) for 4 days to determine PA. The time (min) and percentage (%) of time spent in light, moderate and vigorous PA (MVPA) was determined using specific cut-points for counts per minute related to 3–5 year olds. Of the sample, none of the children met the UK recommended 180 min or more of PA per day. A significant difference ($P < 0.05$) was observed between the amount of time that preschool children spent in sedentary behaviours on weekdays (91.9%) compared to weekend days (96.9%). During weekdays and weekend days, 6.3% and 2.0% of time was spent in MVPA, respectively. Therefore, a substantial proportion of British preschool children's day is spent in sedentary behaviours, with less MVPA accrued during the weekend. Regular engagement during the weekdays provides opportunities to accrue PA, which may not be present on weekend days.

Keywords: physical activity; preschool children; health promotion

1. Introduction

Physical activity (PA) during preschool years is critical to a child's development and overall health and well-being [1,2]; therefore, it is important to integrate PA into early childhood [3,4]. In 2016, over 41 million children worldwide under the age of 5 years were estimated to be overweight [5]. Childhood obesity is an increasing public health concern [6] and weight gained by the age of 5 years has been reported as a predictor of being overweight in adulthood [7]. Physical activity levels and sedentary behaviours of children in the UK have been viewed as 'obesogenic' [8,9], with habitual PA declining over recent years and sedentary behaviour being the dominant state of children's PA levels during their preschool day [4,10–12]. Although studies have examined PA in children aged 5 years and above, fewer studies have been conducted with preschool children. This limited evidence base in UK preschool children's PA levels is therefore a cause for concern.

It has been recommended that preschool children in the UK should ideally be participating in at least 180 min of PA per day [13–15]. Studies have discovered that preschool children spend the majority of their day in sedentary behaviours and a low proportion of their day in moderate to vigorous PA (MVPA) (<15%) [10,16,17]. Of children aged between 2 and 4 years in England, only about one in 10 meet the recommendations of at least 180 min of PA per day [18,19]. It has been reported that children engaged in 7.7 min of MVPA per hour at preschool [20]. Therefore, in accordance with Pate et al. [20], if a child, for example, attends preschool for 8 h, they would only engage in ~1 h of MVPA and it is unlikely they would participate in a further 2 h of PA outside of preschool. However, no study has systematically checked to see whether there is a difference in physical activity between weekdays, when the child attends preschool, and weekend days, when the child is influenced more by their home environment. O'Dwyer et al. [21] reported that there were discrete periods during the after-preschool hours and at the weekend when PA levels were low, yet children who attended preschool for full days engaged in 11.1 min MVPA less than those attending for half days, suggesting that the preschool environment is related to decreased PA. That said, studies have shown that PA in preschoolers differs over the course of the day and the week in countries such as Sweden, England and Denmark [21–24], with some studies reporting that preschool children are more often physically active on weekend days than on weekdays in Australia and England, for example [21,25], while others found that preschool children undertook more total PA and MVPA during preschool hours in Sweden, Denmark, England and Finland [22,24,26,27]. Therefore, additional research is required to identify any potential differences in PA between weekdays and weekend days in preschool children.

The accurate measurement of PA is fundamental in evaluating the effectiveness of interventions and understanding relationships between PA and health [28]. Measuring habitual PA accurately is beneficial when observing the frequency and distribution of PA in preschool children and identifying the amount of PA that could influence their health. The objective monitoring of PA is important and accelerometers have become a reliable and valid way of estimating children's PA [29,30], whilst also showing promise in monitoring preschool children's PA. Accelerometers are an appropriate objective measure in terms of validity, reliability and practicality as a method for the measurement of intensity, duration and frequency of movement for sedentary behaviour and habitual PA in 3–5 year olds [1,31–33]. Accelerometers can be set at different sampling intervals, with some studies being set at one-minute intervals [1,34]. However, one-minute sampling intervals may mask the short intermittent bursts of activity that are representative of young children and therefore shorter sampling intervals have been recommended [20,35]. As very few studies have used objective monitoring of PA via accelerometery in preschool children, then further research is required to examine the intensity of PA that these children participate in on weekdays in preschool and at the weekend.

This is the first study to compare PA levels between week and weekend days, using objective measurements in the form of the newly calibrated GENEActiv accelerometer cut-points for preschool children in the UK. This study aims to determine whether the intensity and duration of PA varies between weekdays and weekend days.

2. Materials and Methods

2.1. Participants and Data Collection

Participants in this study were preschool aged children from 11 preschools in North Warwickshire, England. This study was completed in the Nuneaton and Bedworth Borough, which is in the top 10% of the most deprived Super Output Area's in England on the Index of Multiple Deprivation (IMD) and is ranked as the 111th most deprived Local Authority District out of 326 in England [36]. Ethics approval (P45654) was granted by the Faculty of Health and Life Sciences Ethics Committee, Coventry University and parental consent was obtained. The participants were a convenience sample and included 185 preschool children (99 boys, 86 girls), aged 3–4 years, from a deprived area.

2.2. Anthropometric Assessment

Height was measured to the nearest mm, in bare or sock feet, using a standard portable stadiometer (Leicester height measure, Leicester, UK). Body mass was measured to the nearest 0.1 kg using portable weighing scales (Tanita scales, Tokyo, Japan); the children were lightly dressed (t-shirt and light trousers/skirt) and barefoot or in socks. The measurements were repeated twice and the average score was recorded. Body mass index (BMI) was calculated as kg/m^2 and weight status was categorised as overweight/obese or normal weight using standardised international cut-points [37].

2.3. Assessment of Physical Activity

Daily total PA was measured using a GENEActiv waveform triaxial accelerometer (ActivInsights Ltd., Kimbolton, UK). The accelerometer measured at 10 epochs (s) and a sample frequency of 100 Hz, so as to enable an accurate assessment of the intermittent activities of preschool children [38–40]. The GENEA accelerometer was attached using a watch strap and positioned over the dorsal aspect of the right wrist, midway between the radial and ulnar styloid process. Accelerometers worn on the wrist are more convenient to wear and lead to greater compliance during prolonged wearing when assessing habitual activity [41]. The participants wore the accelerometers for four consecutive days; this included two weekdays in the setting and two weekend days. Each child was required to wear the accelerometer for a minimum of 6 h per day to be included in the study, although it was preferred that they wore them at all times. All children received a letter to take home describing how and when they should wear the GENEActiv accelerometers. Non-wear time was defined as 90-minute windows of consecutive zero or nonzero counts [42]. "Nonzero" counts are caused by artefactual accelerometer movements during non-wear periods—for example, accidental movement of the accelerometer, such as the device being nudged when on a bedside table [42]. The 90-minute window was chosen as this was found to better predict time spent in sedentary behaviours and PA levels [42]. This said, Esliger et al. [43] suggested that a period of 20 min of consecutive zero counts is appropriate for children, as motionless bouts of ≥20 min are biologically implausible. However, it was reported that this low threshold causes an unrealistically high number of non-wear periods [44]. Therefore, it was recommended to use 90 minute consecutive zero counts, as this prevents the overestimation of non-wear time and the underestimation of sedentary behaviours in overweight to obese children [42]. The amount of wear time and percentage (%) of wear time that each child spent in different intensities of PA was calculated for weekdays and weekend days. It is recommended that four days, including one weekend day, is appropriate for measuring habitual PA [45]. Given the logistics of ensuring that children aged 3 years of age wore the accelerometer for the whole monitoring period, participants were included in the final data analysis providing they had worn the accelerometer for 3 days (when in the setting and at the weekend) and for a minimum of six hours each day, similar to previous research [46–48]. Of the 185 sample, 178 children's accelerometer data were recorded; data for seven children were not useable. This was due to the children either not wearing the GENEActiv accelerometers or technical difficulties with the accelerometers or recording of the data. The final sample included in the analysis was 178 children (95 boys, 83 girls), aged 3–4 years. Only four out of the 178 participants were full-time; the remainder were part-time nursery attendees.

For each of the epochs (number of seconds), movement data (activity counts) were added and logged; these were then processed and analysed. Accumulated activity counts were categorised in terms of intensity such as sedentary behaviour, light, moderate and vigorous PA [1]. Cut-points for sedentary behaviour, light PA and moderate and vigorous PA were used to determine the PA intensity of the preschool children. The cut-points used were determined specifically for children aged 4–5 years using GENEA accelerometers, albeit they were calibrated in a laboratory-based study; they are the most relevant cut-points for the preschool children's age in this study (3–4 years) as they are the closest cut-points that are calibrated and reported in the literature [49]. The difference in age should have very little impact on the results, as they are as closely aligned in age as possible and 4 year olds/preschool children have been used for the calibration and ultimately are assessed in this study. The preschool children in the laboratory-based study that was used to determine cut-points for this current study completed six activities, which ranged from lying supine to running. They wore the GENEA accelerometers on both their left and right wrists and used a Cortex mask for gas analysis; VO$_2$ data were used to assess criterion validity [49]. The cut-points determined were as follows: dominant hand <8.1 cpm for sedentary activity, 8.1–9.3 cpm for light activity and 9.3+ cpm for moderate and vigorous PA. For the non-dominant hand, the cut-points were <5.3 cpm for sedentary activity, 5.3–8.6 cpm for light activity and 8.6+ cpm for moderate and vigorous PA [49]. On the accelerometers, the 'Epoch Converter' creates epochs of 1, 5, 10, 15, 30 or 60 s; the means that for each parameter, the Sum Vector Magnitude is calculated for each epoch [50]. Children were classified as either meeting (sufficiently active) or not meeting (insufficiently active) the requirement of 180 min per day of PA for 0–5 year olds.

2.4. Statistical Analysis

The percentage of time in sedentary behaviour, light PA and MVPA was determined, as was the mean amount of time (min) spent in sedentary behaviour, light PA and MVPA, during week and weekend days. Each data set was tested for skewness and kurtosis. Arcsine or inverse data transformation techniques were then used on any data set that did not have a normal distribution, as follows: mean time sedentary for the week and weekend (arcsine transformation); MVPA at the weekend (inverse transformation); percentage time for sedentary behaviour at the weekend (inverse transformation); and MVPA at the weekend (inverse transformation). Any differences in PA due to sex or day of the week were analysed using a series (separate ANCOVA for each category of PA) of 2 (weekday vs. weekend) × 2 (sex) repeated measures analysis of covariance (ANCOVA) controlling for wear time. The Statistical Package for Social Sciences (Version 22, SPSS Inc., Chicago, Ill, USA) was used for statistical analysis and the alpha level was set a priori at $P = 0.05$.

3. Results

Descriptive characteristics, including mean time (min) spent in the different intensities of PA during the week and weekend days, are summarised in Table 1. Of the sample, none of the 178 children met the UK recommended 180 min or more of PA (light, moderate and vigorous intensity) per day. Two, circa 1%, of the children did meet the 180 mins on one of their days, but not on all days.

Table 1. Children's descriptive characteristics. Data represent mean ± SD, $n = 178$.

Characteristics		Values
Age (years)		3.4 ± 0.5
Mass (kg)		16.8 ± 2.5
Height (cm)		101.7 ± 4.8
Body mass index (kg/m^2)		16.3 ± 1.9
Waist circumference (cm)		55.0 ± 3.9
Mean wear time (min) during the week		572.0 ± 99.0
Mean wear time (min) during the weekend		581.0 ± 126.0
Mean sedentary behaviour (min) during the week		527.0 ± 94.0
Mean sedentary behaviour (min) during the weekend		565.0 ± 117.0
Mean light physical activity (PA) (min) during the week		10.0 ± 15.0
Mean light PA (min) during the weekend		7.0 ± 10.0
Mean moderate and vigorous PA (MVPA) (min) during the week		36.0 ± 22.0
Mean moderate and vigorous PA (min) during the weekend		12.0 ± 9.0
Sedentary behaviour (%) during the week		91.9 ± 4.3
Sedentary behaviour (%) during the weekend		96.9 ± 2.0
Light PA (%) during the week		1.8 ± 2.4
Light PA (%) during the weekend		1.1 ± 1.5
MVPA (%) during the week		6.3 ± 3.6
MVPA (%) during the weekend		2.0 ± 1.6
Met PA guidelines of at least 180 min per day total PA (%)	Sufficiently Active	0
	Insufficiently Active	100

Preschool children respectively spent 91.9% and 1.8% of time in sedentary behaviour and light PA on weekdays, and 96.9% and 1.1% of time in sedentary behaviour and light PA at the weekend. During weekdays and weekend days, 6.3% and 2.0% of time was spent in moderate and vigorous PA, respectively. The percentage (%) of daily time spent in different intensities of PA during weekday and weekends for preschool children can be viewed in Figure 1.

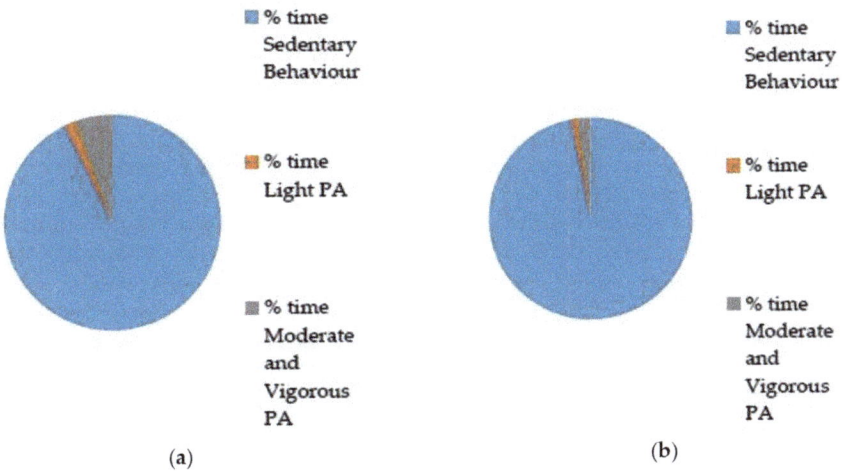

Figure 1. Percentage (%) daily time spent in different intensities of physical activity. (a) Weekdays and (b) weekends for 178 preschool children.

There was a significant difference in the percentage of time (relative) spent in sedentary behaviour between week and weekend days ($P < 0.05$), yet no differences were found between week and weekend days for light or MVPA (Figure 1). There was a significantly smaller mean time in minutes spent in sedentary PA (mean difference = 91.874, $P = 0.001$) during weekdays compared to weekends. This pattern was reversed for moderate and vigorous PA (mean difference = 4.545, $P = 0.001$), with a larger mean time spent in vigorous PA during weekdays compared to weekend days. Wear time had no effect on PA, as there was no significant interaction between wear time and weekday (F = 1.308, $P = 0.257$) or between wear time and weekend day (F = 1.107, $P = 0.297$) for the significant difference reported for the percentage of time (relative) in sedentary behaviour. Sex had no significant effect on any PA intensity (all $P > 0.05$).

4. Discussion

The current study sought to compare PA levels of preschool children between weekdays and weekend days, and the key finding of this study is that there are significant differences in PA between weekdays and weekend days. Of particular note, more than 90% of the time during both weekdays and weekend days was spent in sedentary behaviour. Additionally, this study found that none of the children were considered 'sufficiently active', failing to participate in the UK recommended level of at least 180 min of light PA and MVPA per day of total PA for health. As zero preschool children in this study reported meeting the PA guidelines, this is a major concern, especially as the children were struggling to achieve 60 min of total PA. As the majority of this sample (98%) were part-time preschool children, this could be reflective of this specific preschool child. The children in this study spent time in both the preschool setting and with their parents, in the home environment. It would be pertinent to assess preschool children who are full-time, to ascertain if this provides a similar or different outcome in their PA levels. This would be influential in identifying whether the results of this study are reflective of British preschool children, or if the time children spent in preschool affects their PA levels.

Studies have shown that parents have a significant impact on PA in their preschool children on week and weekend days [51–54]. Therefore, other explanations for the differences in sedentary behaviour between the week and weekend days could be a result of parents displaying higher sedentary behaviours when they are with their children, and children who are exposed to these behaviours copy them during weekend days [55]. This is supported by Sigmundová et al. [56], who found that children from both urban and rural populations had a stronger significant association with sedentary behaviour during weekend days as compared to weekdays. Moore et al. [57] discovered that middle-class American children aged 4–7 years old (incorporating the preschool years), who have one physically active parent, had a relative odds ratio of their child being active between 2.0 (mother) and 3.5 (father). However, if both parents were active then the relative odds ratio was 5.8, with no difference reported between week versus weekend day. Sigmundová et al. [56] monitored children from both urban and rural areas, and discovered that if mothers are more active, then their children are more likely to be more physically active. This was observed to be significant only on weekend days. We do not know the activity patterns of the parents of the children who took part in the present study, but this may have been a contributing factor to the sedentary behaviour patterns that were reported.

A second key finding of this present study is that there are differences in the percentage of time spent in different intensities of PA between weekdays and weekend days for preschool children. During weekdays, the children spent significantly less time in sedentary behaviours (91.9% vs. 96.9%), when compared to weekends. This finding was recorded using the right wrist, which in this study was the dominant hand for 169 of the children (91.4% of the sample). This finding contradicts research by Vásquez et al. [58] in Chilean children (North of Santiago City), who objectively measured PA via a Tritrac-R3D research ergometer and reported that preschool children spent more time in sedentary activities in day-care centres (week vs. weekend) and the children were more active at home at weekends. These differences were also linked with the children's diet and it was discovered that the energy balance was appropriate during the week, as the energy intake in the preschools was reduced. This could explain the differences, as the day-care settings were providing less energy intake; therefore, the children may have been less inclined to be active. Equally, these findings could have been representative of the cultural background, geographical location or differences in the method used for objective measurement of the children involved. A further reason for potential differences between the sedentary behaviours of preschool children during the week and weekend days could be attributed to the time that children spend watching television or playing on computer games, smart phones/tablets (screen time). Previous research has shown that Australian preschool children from different socio-economic backgrounds whose parents limit television viewing spent significantly less time in sedentary behaviours [59]. A study of preschool children from a mixed socio-economic area in the southwest of England reported that 12% of boys and 8% of girls watched ≥2 hours of TV each weekday, compared to 45% of boys and 43% of girls who watched ≥2 h a day on weekend days [60]. The amount of screen time that children in this current study participated in could have been a contributing factor to the differences in time spent in sedentary behaviours during week and weekend days. Parental influence on PA during weekend days may therefore be an important factor that requires greater attention by public health professionals; this could be a result of parents lacking an understanding of appropriate PA to deliver to their children, or a lack of time. Despite this, the extant literature on parental influence on PA levels in British preschool children is scarce. Additional work is required on this topic, in the context of weekday to weekend day variations in children's PA. Equally, the intensity levels of PA of preschool children could be improved through interventions, both in preschools and at home with parents.

Research has reported PA levels and sedentary time as being highly varied and inconsistent between studies across different countries, making it hard to determine preschool children's true PA levels and sedentary behaviour [61]. Reilly [12] measured PA levels from studies over the period of 2000–2008 and discovered that sedentary behaviour was particularly high. However, more recently, in a data collection period from 2006–2009 and a 7 month data collection period in the year 2013, it was reported that 100% of UK preschool children met the recommend daily PA guidelines [22,23]. The current data from this study show that a substantial proportion of each day is spent in sedentary behaviour in British preschool children from a deprived area. This finding has important public health implications around the excessively high sedentary behaviours displayed by preschool children in the UK and therefore provides a clear indication that interventions aiming to convert sedentary behaviours into light or MVPA are required. These data were obtained across a wide measurement period and across all seasons and therefore provide a spread of representative data for the whole of the year. However, this study did not assess each child at different points throughout the year, as it is very labour-intensive and demanding to assess PA in preschool children at one time point and then assess them again across different seasons, and would likely lead to much higher attrition. Therefore, this study did not consider seasonal adjustments. However, future research may consider this, to identify if preschool children are more active in the summer months in England, when compared to the cold environment in the winter months, similar to the results found in 437 preschool children in America [62]. However, this was in contrast to a study of 214 children aged 3–5 years in America, which reported no differences in PA levels between the summer and autumn months [63]. Moreover, further studies in Sweden and America [64,65] also found no variation according to the season of measurement in preschool children. As none of these studies were conducted in England, future research into the seasonal variation of PA in England would be beneficial.

The amount of time spent in different intensities of PA was found to vary between weekdays and weekends, with less moderate and vigorous PA accrued during weekends. However, MVPA was very limited in both parts of the week. Such a finding might be suggestive that regular engagement in the preschool environment provides greater opportunities to accrue PA, which may not be present in the home setting. The light intensity minutes were very low during both the week and weekend days. The wrist-worn accelerometers may not be very precise at detailing light ambulation, where playing with Lego®was at the top end of the sedentary category. Therefore, future research to determine the accuracy of the light PA classifications would be beneficial. Similar research using Actigraphs has shown that using the cut-point of 160 cpm to distinguish light intensity from sedentary behaviours is questionable [66]. It is believed that this threshold may misclassify sedentary behaviours such as seated play and crafts as light intensity, which would cause an overestimation of total PA minutes and underestimate the steps per day [66] that are required to achieve the daily UK 180 minutes of recommended PA. This is a current problem, as there is no consensus on the optimal cut-points for distinguishing sedentary from light PA in preschool children [56]. Also, the cut-points used for light intensity PA in this study were taken from laboratory-derived tasks that were constant in nature, whereas the real-life activities of preschool children are more varied and intermittent. This may have made it more difficult to differentiate light PA from sedentary behaviour, as the determination is dependent on the cut-point used. However, this is a feature of most of the research using accelerometers to classify/assess PA [66,67]. Therefore, it could be suggested that the cut-points used in this study were too conservative, however, as they are the only cut-points related to preschool children specifically for the GENEActiv accelerometers, then they were the most appropriate to have adopted.

Using wrist-worn accelerometers can be logistically and practically challenging with preschool children [31], as the accelerometer can sometimes be regarded as uncomfortable or an annoyance when worn for long periods of time, thus questioning the appropriateness of the accelerometer for preschool children. In the current study, although a cut-off of 6 h per day was employed for inclusion in the data analysis, the participants exceeded this value with total mean wear time per day for all days, which was over 577 min (>9.6 h). The mean wear time for weekdays was 573 min (9.6 h) and that for weekend days was 581 min (>9.7 h). We took this to be an indication that the majority of the children in this study were comfortable wearing the accelerometers. It could be questioned whether <600 min/day (10 h) is a true representation of a preschool child's whole day (24 h). It would be beneficial for future research to measure PA for a greater duration, for example 12 hours, to see if this affects the total PA in a day, in terms of less sedentary behaviours and more MVPA. As mentioned, it could be questioned whether wearing the accelerometer on the wrist is suitable for preschool children. Research has looked at the difference between wearing a wrist and hip accelerometer on preschool children and one study in Scotland found that wrist-worn accelerometers provided a valid estimate of total physical activity, whereas hip-worn accelerometers showed a reasonable agreement to cut-points [68]. This was supported by a study in Stockholm, Sweden, which similarly monitored preschool children and found that wrist-worn accelerometers performed more accurately when assessing time spent in sedentary, light activity and MVPA, when compared to hip-worn accelerometers [69]. In terms a study by Johannsson et al. [69], however, there were stark differences between the mean (SD) counts measured over 5 s for wrist and hip activity, with the vector magnitude (a combined measure of the three axes, x, y and z) when watching a cartoon measuring 91 (73) for the wrist and 14 (15) for the hip, and when dancing, the 1093 (330) was measured for the wrist and 396 (148) for the hip. These are large contrasts, highlighting that where the accelerometers are worn is an important factor to be considered. This present study had the preschool children wearing them on their wrist, which, in accordance with other studies [68,69], is the more accurate and valid place to wear them when using the vector magnitude measure, as opposed to the vertical axis measure.

Although the current study successfully used accelerometery as an objective monitoring tool in preschool children, some limitations should also be considered. Some of the accelerometers failed to record data; this manufacturer problem caused no data to be recorded for seven participants. GENEActiv accelerometers worn at the wrist may not be capable of detailing light ambulation precisely, as possibly indicated by the low levels of light PA reported. Equally, wrist-worn accelerometers in young children may also impact the light intensity PA data; however, the research does appear to show that the location, whether at the wrist or hip, has no significant effect on the PA levels reported [70,71]. As previously stated, the preschool children were assessed once in a season and not across all seasons. Although children were assessed throughout different seasons, which provided representative data, the lack of assessment of each child in all seasons should be considered a limitation of the study. The preschool children that were monitored were drawn from a deprived part of the UK. It has been reported that the prevalence of obesity amongst 4–5 year olds in the most deprived 10% of England is approximately double the levels of the least deprived 10% of England [72]. In this current study, 10.8% (20 out of 185) were considered obese. Low socio-economic status (SES) children face greater barriers to becoming physically active and, as they age, low SES individuals have higher rates of obesity and associated comorbidities [73]. Additionally, people from lower SES groups predominantly live in areas that do not support walking and cycling [74]. This viewpoint suggests that deprived areas do not facilitate PA as effectively as other areas and, as such, people living in deprived areas may not participate in PA as frequently. This said, further research comparing both high and low socio-economic status groups would be welcome to extend the literature on preschool children. Understanding the levels of PA in this group is useful to allow for the planning of early interventions to improve current and future health.

5. Conclusions

The current study is the first to objectively compare PA levels between weekdays and weekend days in preschool children in the UK using GENEActiv accelerometers, and one of the first to report objectively monitored PA levels of preschool children from deprived areas in the UK. The results of this study suggest that none of the preschool children in this sample achieved the UK recommended guidelines of PA for health. Additionally, and of great concern, it was found that preschool children spend 90% of their time engaged in sedentary behaviours. This study indicates that preschool children participate in more MVPA during weekdays compared to weekend days; however, participation in MVPA was minimal throughout the week. This information can help to promote future interventions that focus on enhancing PA and encouraging participation in LPA and MVPA during both week and weekend days, so as to improve physical development and a healthy weight status in preschool children.

Author Contributions: C.M.P.R.: conception and design of the study, data acquisition (participant measurements), analysis of the data, preparation of the tables and figures, preparation of the manuscript, finding relevant references and final approval of the manuscript. M.J.D.: conception and design of the study, analysis of the data, writing—review and editing and final approval of the manuscript. R.S.J.: analysis of the data, writing—review and editing.

Funding: This research received no external funding.

Conflicts of Interest: The authors declare no conflict of interest.

References

1. Adolph, A.L.; Puyau, M.R.; Vohra, F.A.; Nicklas, T.A.; Zakeri, I.F.; Butte, N.F. Validation of unixal and triaxal accelerometers for the assessment of physical activity in preschool children. *J. Phys. Act. Health* **2012**, *9*, 944–953. [CrossRef] [PubMed]
2. Esliger, D.W.; Tremblay, M.S. Physical activity and inactivity profiling: The next generation. *Can. J. Public Health* **2007**, *98*, S195–S207. [CrossRef] [PubMed]
3. Strong, W.B.; Malina, R.M.; Blimkie, C.J.; Daniels, S.R.; Dishman, R.K.; Gutin, B.B.; Hergenroeder, A.C.; Must, A.; Nixon, P.A.; Pivarnik, J.M.; et al. Evidence based physical activity for school-age youth. *J. Pediatr.* **2005**, *146*, 732–737. [CrossRef] [PubMed]
4. Tucker, P. The physical activity levels of preschool-aged children: A systematic review. *Early Child. Res. Q.* **2008**, *23*, 547–558. [CrossRef]
5. World Health Organization. Global Strategy on Diet, Physical Activity and Health. Childhood Overweight and Obesity. Available online: https://www.who.int/dietphysicalactivity/childhood/en/ (accessed on 16 May 2019).
6. de Onis, M.; Blössner, M. Prevalence and trends of overweight among preschool children in developing countries. *Am. J. Clin. Nutr.* **2000**, *72*, 1032–1039. [CrossRef] [PubMed]
7. Guo, S.S.; Chumlea, W.C. Tracking of body mass index in children in relation to overweight in adulthood. *Am. J. Clin. Nutr.* **1999**, *70*, S145–S148. [CrossRef] [PubMed]
8. Reilly, J.J.; Jackson, D.M.; Montgomery, C.; Kelly, L.A.; Slater, C.; Grant, S.; Paton, J.Y. Total energy expenditure and physical activity in young Scottish children: Mixed longitudinal study. *Lancet* **2004**, *363*, 211–212. [CrossRef]
9. Reilly, J.J.; Armstrong, J.; Dorosty, A.R.; Emmett, P.M.; Ness, A.; Rogers, I.; Steer, C.; Sheriff, A. Early life risk factors for childhood obesity: Cohort study. *Br. Med. J.* **2005**, *330*, 1357–1362. Available online: http://www.bmj.com/content/330/7504/1357 (accessed on 24 October 2012).
10. Jackson, D.M.; Reilly, J.J.; Kelly, L.A.; Montgomery, C.; Grant, S.; Paton, J.Y. Objectively measured physical activity in a representative sample of 3- to 4-year old children. *Obes. Res.* **2003**, *11*, 420–425. [CrossRef] [PubMed]
11. Raustorp, A.; Pagels, P.; Boldemann, C.; Cosco, N.; Söderström, M.; Mårtensson, F. Accelerometer measured level of physical activity indoors and outdoors during preschool time in Sweden and the United States. *J. Phys. Act. Health* **2012**, *9*, 801–808. [CrossRef] [PubMed]
12. Reilly, J.J. Low levels of objectively measured physical activity in pre-schoolers in childcare. *Med. Sci. Sports Exerc.* **2010**, *42*, 502–507. [CrossRef]
13. Department of Health. Physical Activity Guidelines for Early Years (under 5s)—for Children Who Are Capable of Walking. Available online: https://www.gov.uk/government/publications/uk-physical-activity-guidelines (accessed on 18 May 2016).
14. National Association for Sport and Physical Education. Active Start: A Statement of Physical Activity Guidelines for Children from Birth to Age 5, 2nd Edition. Available online: https://www.columbus.gov/uploadedFiles/Public_Health/Content_Editors/Planning_and_Performance/Healthy_Children_Healthy_Weights/NASPE%20Active%20Start.pdf (accessed on 18 March 2016).
15. Reilly, J.J.; Okely, A.D.; Almond, L.; Cardon, G.; Prosser, L.; Hubbard, J. Making the Case for UK Physical Activity Guidelines for Early Years: Recommendations and Draft Summary statements Based on the Current Evidence. Working Paper. Available online: http://www.google.co.uk/url?sa=t&rct=j&q=&esrc=s&frm=1&source=web&cd=2&sqi=2&ved=0CCoQFjAB&url=http%3A%2F%2Fwww.paha.org.uk%2FFile%2FIndex%2Fe53f5ad2--85ed-443b-ae85--9f1d00fc9ee4&ei=UTSRUOKLJsq50QXQ4IDoBw&usg=AFQjCNEhmTG6oSxvGXpFWK5-pAdV1Kn0ww&sig2=DkO1rbQBs6MWNMPp6rHjyw (accessed on 19 December 2012).

16. Montgomery, C.; Reilly, J.J.; Jackson, D.M.; Kelly, L.A.; Slater, C.; Paton, J.Y.; Grant, S. Relation between physical activity and energy expenditure in a representative sample of young children. *Am. J. Clin. Nutr.* **2004**, *80*, 591–596. [CrossRef] [PubMed]
17. Pate, R.R.; McIver, K.; Dowda, M.; Brown, W.H.; Addy, C. Directly observed physical activity levels in preschool children. *J. Sch. Health* **2008**, *78*, 438–444. [CrossRef] [PubMed]
18. Health and Social Care Information Centre. Health Survey for England—2012. Available online: http://www.hscic.gov.uk/catalogue/PUB13218 (accessed on 10 July 2016).
19. National Health Service (NHS) Digital. Health Survey for England. 2015. Available online: http://www.content.digital.nhs.uk/catalogue/PUB22610/HSE2015-Child-phy-act.pdf (accessed on 12 April 2017).
20. Pate, R.R.; Pfeiffer, K.A.; Trost, S.G.; Ziegler, P.; Dowda, M. Physical activity among children attending preschools. *Pediatrics* **2004**, *114*, 1258–1263. [CrossRef] [PubMed]
21. O'Dwyer, M.; Fairclough, S.J.; Ridgers, N.D.; Knowles, Z.R.; Foweather, L.; Stratton, G. Patterns of Objectively Measured Moderate-to-Vigorous Physical Activity in Preschool Children. *J. Phys. Act. Health* **2014**, *11*, 1233–1238. [CrossRef] [PubMed]
22. Hesketh, K.R.; McMinn, A.M.; Ekelund, U.; Sharp, S.J.; Collings, P.J.; Harvey, N.C.; Godfrey, K.M.; Inskip, H.M.; Cooper, C.; van Sluijs, E.M.F. Objectively measured physical activity in four-year-old British children: A cross-sectional analysis of activity patterns segmented across the day. *Int. J. Behav. Nutr. Phys. Act.* **2014**, *11*, 1. [CrossRef] [PubMed]
23. Hesketh, K.R.; Griffin, S.J.; van Sluijs, E.M.F. UK preschool-aged children's physical activity levels in childcare and at home: A cross-sectional exploration'. *Int. J. Behav. Nutr. Phys. Act.* **2015**, *12*, 123. [CrossRef] [PubMed]
24. Møller, N.C.; Christensen, L.B.; Mølgaard, C.; Ejlerskov, K.T.; Pfeiffer, K.A.; Michaelsen, F. Descriptive analysis of preschool physical activity and sedentary behaviours—A cross sectional study of 3-year olds nested in the SKOT cohort. *BMC Public Health* **2017**, *17*, 613. [CrossRef] [PubMed]
25. Hinkley, T.; Salmon, J.; Okely, A.D.; Crawford, D.; Hesketh, K. Preschoolers' physical activity, screen time, and compliance with recommendations. *Med. Sci. Sports Exerc.* **2012**, *44*, 458–465. [CrossRef] [PubMed]
26. Berglind, D.; Tynelius, P. Objectively measured physical activity patterns, sedentary time and parent-reported screen-time across the day in four-year-old Swedish children. *BMC Public Health* **2017**, *18*, 69. [CrossRef] [PubMed]
27. Soini, A.; Tammelin, T.; Sääkslahti, A.; Watt, A.; Villberg, J.; Kettunen, T.; Mehtälä, A.; Poskiparta, M. Seasonal and daily variation in physical activity among three-year-old Finnish preschool children. *Early Child Dev. Care* **2014**, *184*, 589–601. [CrossRef]
28. Haskell, W.L.; Lee, I.L.; Pate, R.R.; Powell, K.E.; Blair, S.N.; Franklin, B.A.; Macera, C.A.; Heath, G.W.; Thompson, P.D.; Bauman, A. Physical activity and public health: Updated recommendation for adults from the American College of Sports Medicine and the American Heart Association. *Med. Sci. Sports Exerc.* **2007**, *39*, 1423–1434. [CrossRef] [PubMed]
29. Pate, R.R.; Almeida, M.J.; McIver, K.L.; Pfeiffer, K.A.; Dowda, M. Validation and calibration of an accelerometer in preschool children. *Obesity* **2006**, *14*, 2000–2006. [CrossRef] [PubMed]
30. Phillips, L.R.S.; Parfitt, G.; Rowlands, A.V. Calibration of the GENEA accelerometer for assessment of physical activity intensity in children. *J. Sci. Med. Sport* **2013**, *16*, 124–128. [CrossRef] [PubMed]
31. Cliff, D.P.; Okely, A.D.; Smith, L.M.; McKeen, K. Relationships between fundamental movement skills and objectively measured physical activity in preschool children. *Pediatr. Exerc. Sci.* **2009**, *21*, 436–449. [CrossRef] [PubMed]
32. Reilly, J.J.; Coyle, J.; Kelly, L.; Burke, G.; Grant, S.; Paton, J.Y. An objective method for measurement of sedentary behaviour in 3- to 4-year olds. *Obes. Res.* **2003**, *11*, 1155–1158. [CrossRef] [PubMed]
33. Westerterp, K.R. Physical activity assessment with accelerometers. *Int. J. Obes. Relat. Met. Disord.* **1999**, *23*, S45–S49. [CrossRef]
34. Evenson, K.R.; Terry, J.W. Assessment of differing definitions of accelerometer non-wear time. *Res. Q. Exerc. Sport* **2009**, *80*, 355–362. [CrossRef] [PubMed]
35. Rowlands, A.V. Accelerometer assessment of physical activity in children: An update. *Pediatr. Exerc. Sci.* **2007**, *19*, 252–266. [CrossRef] [PubMed]
36. Warwickshire Government. Warwickshire Joint Strategic Needs Assessment (JSNA) The Essential Tool to Inform Commissioning. Deprivation in Warwickshire. Available online: http://hwb.warwickshire.gov.uk/warwickshire-people-and-place/deprivation/ (accessed on 21 June 2019).

37. Cole, T.J.; Bellizzi, M.C.; Flegal, K.M.; Dietz, W.H. Establishing a standard definition for children overweight and obesity worldwide: International survey. *BMJ* **2000**, *320*, 1240–1243. [CrossRef] [PubMed]
38. Hasselstrøm, H.; Karlsson, K.M.; Hansen, S.E.; Grønfeldt, V.; Froberg, K.; Andersen, L.B. Peripheral bone mineral density and different intensities of physical activity in children 6–8 years old: The Copenhagen School Child Intervention Study. *Calcif. Tissue Int.* **2007**, *80*, 31–38. [CrossRef] [PubMed]
39. Obeid, J.; Nguyen, T.; Gabel, L.; Timmons, B.W. Physical activity in Ontario preschoolers: Prevalence and measurement issues. *Appl. Physiol. Nutr. Metab.* **2011**, *36*, 291–297. [CrossRef]
40. Vale, V.; Santos, R.; Silva, P.; Soares-Miranda, L.; Mota, J. Preschool Children Physical Activity Measurement: Importance of Epoch Length Choice. *Pédiatr. Exerc. Sci* **2009**, *21*, 413–420. [CrossRef] [PubMed]
41. Zhang, S.; Rowlands, A.V.; Murray, P.; Hurst, T. Physical activity classification using the GENEA wrist-worn accelerometer. *Med. Sci. Sports Exerc.* **2012**, *44*, 742–748. [CrossRef] [PubMed]
42. Choi, L.; Liu, Z.; Matthews, C.E.; Buchowski, M.S. Validation of accelerometer wear and nonwear time classification algorithm. *Med. Sci. Sports Exerc.* **2011**, *43*, 357–364. [CrossRef]
43. Esliger, D.W.; Copeland, J.; Barnes, J.D.; Tremblay, M.S. Standardizing and Optimizing the Use of Accelerometer Data for Free-Living Physical Activity Monitoring. *J. Phys. Act. Health* **2005**, *3*, 366–383. [CrossRef]
44. Chinapaw, M.J.M.; de Niet, M.; Verloigne, M.; De Bourdeaudhuij, I.; Brug, J.; Altenburg, T.M. From sedentary time to sedentary patterns: Accelerometer data reduction decisions in youth. *PLoS ONE* **2014**, *9*, e111205. [CrossRef]
45. Trost, S.G.; Pate, R.R.; Freedson, P.S.; Sallis, J.F.; Taylor, W.C. Using objective physical activity measures with youth: How many days of monitoring are needed? *Med. Sci. Sports Exerc.* **2000**, *32*, 426–431. [CrossRef]
46. Benham-Deal, T. Preschool children's accumulated and sustained physical activity. *Percept. Mot. Ski.* **2005**, *100*, 443–450. [CrossRef]
47. King, N.; Horrocks, C. *Interviews in Qualitative Research*; Sage: London, UK, 2010.
48. Trost, S.G.; Sirard, J.R.; Dowda, M.; Pfeiffer, K.A.; Pate, R.R. Physical activity in overweight and non-overweight preschool children. *Int. J. Obes. Relat. Metab. Disord.* **2003**, *27*, 834–839. [CrossRef]
49. Roscoe, C.M.P.; James, R.; Duncan, M. Calibration of GENEActiv accelerometer wrist cut-points for the assessment of physical activity intensity of preschool aged children. *Eur. J. Pediatr.* **2017**, *176*, 1093–1098. [CrossRef]
50. GENEActiv. GENEActiv Instructions Manual version 1.2. 2012. Available online: http://www.geneactiv.org/wpcontent/uploads/2014/03/geneactiv_instruction_manual_v1.2.pdf (accessed on 18 January 2018).
51. Hesketh, K.R.; Goodfellow, L.; Ekelund, U.; McMinn, A.M.; Godfrey, K.M.; Inskip, H.M.; Cooper, C.; Harvey, N.C.; van Sluijs, E.M. Activity levels in mothers and their preschool children. *Pediatrics* **2014**, *133*, e973–e980. [CrossRef]
52. Oliver, M.; Schofield, G.M.; Schluter, P.J. Parent influences on preschoolers' objectively assessed physical activity. *J. Sci. Med. Sport* **2010**, *13*, 403–409. [CrossRef]
53. Sigmundová, D.; Sigmund, E.; Badura, P.; Vokáčová, J.; Trhliková, L.; Bucksch, J. Weekday-weekend patterns of physical activity and screen time in parents and their pre-schoolers. *BMC Public Health* **2016**, *16*, 898. [CrossRef]
54. Vollmer, R.L.; Adamsons, K.; Gorin, A.; Foster, J.S.; Mobley, A.R. Investigating the relationship of body mass index, diet quality, and physical activity level between fathers and their preschool-aged children. *J. Acad. Nutr. Diet.* **2015**, *115*, 919–926. [CrossRef]
55. Sigmund, E.; Turoňová, K.; Sigmundová, D.; Přidalová, M. The effect of parent's physical activity and inactivity on their children's physical activity and sitting. *Acta Univ. Palacki. Olomuc. Gymn.* **2008**, *38*, 17–24.
56. Sigmundová, D.; Sigmund, E.; Vokáčová, J.; Kopčáková, J. Parent-child associations in pedometer-determined physical activity and sedentary behaviour on weekdays and weekends in random samples of families in the Czech Republic. *Int. J. Environ. Res. Public Health* **2014**, *11*, 7163–7181. [CrossRef]
57. Moore, L.L.; Lombardi, D.A.; White, M.J.; Campbell, J.L.; Oliveria, S.A.; Ellison, R.C. Influence of parents' physical activity levels on activity levels of young children. *J. Pediatr.* **1991**, *118*, 215–219. [CrossRef]
58. Vasquez, F.; Salazar, G.; Andrade, M.; Vasquez, L.; Diaz, E. Energy balance and physical activity in obese children attending daycare centres. *Eur. J. Clin. Nutr.* **2006**, *60*, 1115–1121. [CrossRef]

59. Hnatiuk, J.A.; Salmon, J.; Campbell, K.J.; Ridgers, N.D.; Hesketh, K.D. Tracking of maternal self-efficacy for limiting young children's television viewing and associations with children's television viewing time: A longitudinal analysis over 15-months. *BMC Public Health* **2015**, *15*, 517. [CrossRef]
60. Jago, R.; Thompson, J.; Sebire, S.; Wood, L.; Pool, L.; Zahra, J.; Lawlor, D. Crosssectional associations between the screen-time of parents and young children: Differences by parent and child gender and day of the week. *Int. J. Behav. Nutr. Phys. Act.* **2014**, *11*, 54. [CrossRef]
61. O'Brien, K.T.; Vanderloo, L.M.; Bruijns, B.A.; Truelove, S.; Tucker, P. Physical activity and sedentary time among preschoolers in centre-based childcare: A systematic review. *Int. J. Behav. Nutr. Phys. Act.* **2018**, *15*, 117. [CrossRef]
62. Rundle, A.; Goldstein, I.F.; Mellins, R.B.; Ashby-Thompson, M.; Hoepner, L.; Jacobson, J.S. Physical Activity and Asthma Symptoms among New York City Head Start Children. *J. Asthma* **2009**, *46*, 803–809. [CrossRef]
63. Finn, K.; Johannsen, N.; Specker, B. Factors associated with physical activity in preschool children. *J. Pediatr.* **2002**, *140*, 81–85. [CrossRef]
64. Bringolf-Isler, B.; Grize, L.; Mader, U.; Ruch, N.; Sennhauser, F.H.; Braun-Fahrlander, C. Assessment of intensity, prevalence and duration of everyday activities in Swiss school children: A cross-sectional analysis of accelerometer and diary data. *Int. J. Behav. Nutr. Phys. Act.* **2009**, *6*, 50. [CrossRef]
65. Burdette, H.L.; Whitaker, R.C.; Daniels, S.R. Parental report of outdoor playtime as a measure of physical activity in preschool-aged children. *Arch. Pediatr. Adolesc. Med.* **2004**, *158*, 353–357. [CrossRef]
66. Vale, S.; Trost, S.G.; Duncan, M.J.; Mota, J. Step based physical activity guidelines for preschool aged children. *Prev. Med.* **2015**, *70*, 78–82. [CrossRef]
67. Kim, Y.; Lee, J.-M.; Peters, B.P.; Gaesser, G.A.; Welk, G.J. Examination of different accelerometer cut-points for assessing sedentary behaviours in children. *PLoS ONE* **2014**, *9*, e90630. [CrossRef]
68. Hislop, J.; Palmer, N.; Anand, P.; Aldin, T. Validity of writs worn accelerometers and comparability sites in estimating physical activity behaviour in preschool children. *Physiol. Meas.* **2016**, *37*, 1701–1714. [CrossRef]
69. Johansson, E.; Larisch, L.-M.; Marcus, C.; Hagströmer, M. Calibration and Validation of a Wrist- and Hip-Worn Actigraph Accelerometer in 4- Year-Old Children. *PLoS ONE* **2016**, *11*, e0162436. [CrossRef]
70. Dieu, O.; Mikulovic, J.; Fardy, P.S.; Bui-Xuan, G.; Beghin, L.; Vanhelst, J. Physical activity using wrist-worn accelerometers: Comparison of dominant and non-dominant wrist. *Clin. Physiol. Funct. Imaging* **2017**, *37*, 525–529. [CrossRef]
71. Rowlands, A.V.; Rennie, K.; Kozarski, R.; Stanley, R.M.; Eston, R.G.; Parfitt, G.C.; Olds, T.S. Children's physical activity assessed with wrist- and hip-worn accelerometers. *Med. Sci. Sports Exerc.* **2014**, *46*, 2308–2316. [CrossRef]
72. Public Health England. NCMP Local Authority Profile. Available online: http://fingertips.phe.org.uk/profile/national-child-measurement-programme/data#gid/8000011/pat/6/ati/101/page/1/par/E12000005/are/E07000219 (accessed on 27 April 2014).
73. National Obesity Observatory. Patterns and Trends in Child Obesity. Available online: http://www.noo.org.uk/slide_sets (accessed on 25 April 2014).
74. The Marmot Review Team. Fair Society, Healthy Lives: Strategic Review of the Health Inequalities in England post-2010: The Marmot Review: London. Available online: https://www.gov.uk/dfid-research-outputs/fair-society-healthy-lives-the-marmot-review-strategic-review-of-health-inequalities-in-england-post-2010 (accessed on 28 March 2016).

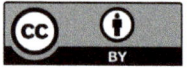

© 2019 by the authors. Licensee MDPI, Basel, Switzerland. This article is an open access article distributed under the terms and conditions of the Creative Commons Attribution (CC BY) license (http://creativecommons.org/licenses/by/4.0/).

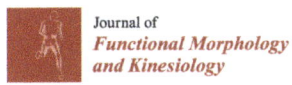

Article

Joint Mobility Protection during the Developmental Age among Free Climbing Practitioners: A Pilot Study

Ludovica Gasbarro [1],[†], Elvira Padua [1],[†], Virginia Tancredi [2], Giuseppe Annino [2], Michela Montorsi [1],[*], Grazia Maugeri [3],[*] and Agata Grazia D'Amico [1]

[1] Department of Human Sciences and Promotion of the Quality of Life, San Raffaele Roma Open University, 00166 Rome, Italy; gasbarroludovica@gmail.com (L.G.); elvira.padua@uniroma5.it (E.P.); agata.damico@uniroma5.it (A.G.D.)
[2] Department of Systems Medicine, University of Rome Tor Vergata, 00166 Rome, Italy; virginia.tancredi@uniroma5.it (V.T.); g_annino@hotmail.com (G.A.)
[3] Section of Anatomy, Histology and Movement Sciences, Department of Biomedical and Biotechnological Sciences, University of Catania, 95123 Catania, Italy
* Correspondence: michela.montorsi@uniroma5.it (M.M.); graziamaugeri@unict.it (G.M.); Tel.: +39-0652-252552 (M.M.); +39-0953-782127 (G.M.)
† These authors contributed equally to this work.

Received: 5 September 2019; Accepted: 10 February 2020; Published: 17 February 2020

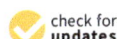

Abstract: Sport-climbing popularity increased intensely over the past years. Particularly, children's and adolescents' interest therein is constantly growing. Despite a large effort in preventing injuries and muscle overloads, a fine-tuned training for each sensitive phase of child development is still needed. The objective of the study was to evaluate an innovative training program aimed at the preservation of joint mobility during the developmental age. This article relies on the results of a steady training program allowing to retain joints integrity among the practice of sport climbing in children. Joint mobility changes have been monitored before and after a one-year training program in fifteen subjects aged between 8 and 18 years. Subjects were divided into three groups depending on age (Turgor Secundus, Proceritas Secunda and Turgor Tertius). The motor tests administered were the sit-and-reach test, coxo-femoral mobility test and scapula–humeral mobility test. Our results showed that one-year training improved joint mobility at each analyzed phase, suggesting that this training program could improve mobility and flexibility. Given the importance of joint mobility preservation for discipline-related injuries prevention and eventually recovering, it is essential to provide a specific training program as a route to approach sport climbing, and even more importantly, at an early age. This work represents a preliminary study in order to demonstrate both efficacy on the joint mobility and the requirement of our playful work to support the global sport-climbing workout.

Keywords: joint mobility; development phases; sport climbing; stretching

---

1. Introduction

In the last decades, rock climbing has become a popular sport among adults, adolescents and children, also since it being included in the 2018 Summer Olympic Youth Games in Buenos Aires and in the Summer Olympic program of the 2020 Games in Tokyo [1,2]. In using only their bare hands and climbing shoes to perform a range of hand and foot holds, athletes climb vertical walls in three disciplines: Speed, with two climbers simultaneously climbing a route on a 15 m wall; Bouldering, with athletes performing in a given time a number of fixed routes on a 4m wall; and Lead, with athletes climbing in a given time a 15 m wall [3]. It is possible to practice it not only outdoor, as now there also are indoor structures; so, this sport is becoming widespread in adults and adolescents, too.

Rock climbing has several benefits on both physical fitness and mental care. In fact, this sport improves strength and endurance [4,5]. A recent study [6] has demonstrated that rock climbing significantly improves muscle power, ability to produce a maximal force in a short time, muscle endurance and skills to perform a continuous muscle work for a long time. This kind of sport also has beneficial effects on depressive disorders due to the positive effect on cognitive control of the physical activity connected to high levels of coordination [7]. It has been demonstrated that only a single rock-climbing session may have a positive effect in major depressive disorder [8].

Due to the increased popularity, the average age of rock climbers is decreasing, and more and more young athletes win medals. Unfortunately, the increased number of young rock climbers involves a major risk of an injury in the developmental age [9].

During climbing very small parts of the hands and feet are in contact with the climbing surface [10–12] and climbers have to support and/or lift their bodies by combining a variety of finger grips with balanced, complex vertical and lateral movements and position holds [13,14]. To guarantee grip and stability, specialized smooth climbing footwear with a sticky rubber sole are used. Although climbing shoes should fit snug without pain, the climbers tend to use smaller sizes, which could cause injuries or foot deformation [15].

Physical activity is essential to maintain good health and guarantee a better quality of life. The major sport-related benefits involve not only the body but also the mind. In fact, physical activity improves motor and cognitive skills, reduces risk for obesity, exerts positive effects on blood pressure and lipidemia, as well as decreasing the risk of depression and other mental disorders [16,17]. However, incorrect or excessive training may lead to adverse effects, including musculoskeletal injuries, recently described in young soccer players, as well as social–occupational dysfunction [18,19]. In particular, in rock climbing the articulations are very solicited and the scientific literature reports injuries in fingers or in shoulders [15,20]. In particular, Garcia et al. [21] examined hands and fingers of young climbers versus a control group of non-climbers and they showed a non-physiological development of fingers. Similarly, another study [22] showed differences in the static scapular position between rock climbers and a control group.

In particularly the developmental age there is a major risk of sprains, strains and fractures with chronicle injuries at the upper extremity and acute injuries at the lower extremity [23]. A survey among rock climbers [24] reports 90% upper extremity injuries, and among these the most common are fingers followed by shoulder/arm and elbow/forearm.

Rock climbing is positively related to increased bone mineral content, weight and mass body [15]. However, for climbers a low body mass index is an ideal anthropometric requirement. Therefore, they perform a restricted diet to maintain a low body weight, by inducing a negative effect on their health and in particular on their bones [25,26]. Moreover, the stresses associated with rock climbing may have the potential to create scapula–humeral or coxo–femoral injuries [22].

Despite the increase in rock-climbing practices and the consequent increase in studies on the benefits or injuries of climbing, little data are available on adolescents.

To envision the development of effective preventative measures for preserving the joint mobility and health of youth practitioners, the aim of this preliminary study was to evaluate the effects of a specific pre-training rock climbing program to be administered to athletes according to their developmental status.

Therefore, in this preliminary study we evaluated an innovative training program to preserve joint mobility during the developmental age. Children were subjected to a steady training program in order to retain joint integrity and to avoid climbing-associated injuries.

2. Materials and Methods

2.1. Subjects

Fifteen subjects aged between 8 and 18 years, working out regularly in sport climbing and joint mobility, were divided into 3 groups consisting of 5 athletes each according to their ages. Turgor Secundus (3 boys and 2 girls; aged between 8 and 10), Proceritas Secunda (2 boys and 3 girls; aged between 12 and 14) and Turgor Tertius (2 boys and 3 girls; aged between 15 and 18).

Table 1 reports the anthropometric characteristics of the athletes, divided in subgroups according to their developmental phase.

Table 1. Characteristics of participants recruited to conduct the present study expressed as mean fold change ± SEM.

Characteristic	TURGOR SECUNDUS (Mean ± SEM)	PROCERITAS SECUNDA (Mean ± SEM)	TURGOR TERTIUS (Mean ± SEM)
Age	8.80 ± 0.37	13.00 ± 0.45	16.60 ± 0.51
Weight	28.80 ± 1.46	49.00 ± 2.97	55.20 ± 3.61
Height	128.60 ± 1.81	160.00 ± 2.98	167.80 ± 3.44
BMI	17.46 ± 1.03	19.15 ± 1.08	19.53 ± 0.73

This study received the consence by the Institutional Research Board of the University San Raffaele of Rome, Italy and all subjects' legal tutors gave written informed consent in respecting the ethical principles of the Declaration of Helsinki. All participants were novices regarding climbing experience.

2.2. Methodology

Knowledge of the main physiological changes and the sensitive phases of development is fundamental for the educator, as on the basis of this information he can develop a program suitable for the child's needs. The sensitive phases of development are periods of growth in which the child will be predisposed to increase some motor skills rather than others. Furthermore, the differential growing of the bones, nervous system and muscles in the different evolutionary phases must be taken into consideration in the programming to avoid injuries and the onset of paramorphism.

Our study was conducted for 12 months, and during this experimental period the climbing training program was carried out according to the coach's training plan. Children worked out twice a week for 90 min divided as follow: 15 min for stretching, 20 min for specific training to improve joint mobility and 55 min for climbing.

Joint mobility variation was assessed over a one-year training period. All the measurements were performed at baseline (time 0; start measurement) and repeated at the end of the training period (time 1; after 12 months) in order to evaluate scapula–humeral and coxo–femoral joint mobility and spine flexibility. The measures recorded in time 0 were considered our control data and the measures obtained at the end of training program were compared to data recorded in time 0 in order to calculate the improvement of joint mobility for each group.

Tests have been performed as follows:

Sit-and-reach test: Participants sat on the floor with legs extended, backs straight and feet resting on a cube with a graduated wooden board above it. The participants are asked to slide their hands above the wooden board, keeping the knee extended [27].

Hip joint mobility: Participants are sitting with their back against the wall, slowly reaching the maximum opening of their hips. The measurement is then taken between the inner ankles [28].

Scapulo–humeral mobility test (measurement of shoulder mobility): Participants are in an upright position, holding a stick, bringing the arms outstretched behind the trunk and reaching the starting position without bending the arms. Then, the minimum distance between the hands while the subject is holding the stick was measured [29].

2.3. Training Regime

Participants of the three experimental groups underwent a specific training program 2 times/week, performing 15 min of general warm-up before training. The specific training program for each phase was done for 20 min before rock climbing.

According to each phase, the following training methods were proposed in order to improve joint mobility.

The Turgor Secundus phase: Obstacle course on wall bars (Figure 1) to preserve a good degree of flexibility and to practice the typical positions of sport climbing:

Exercise 1: The aim was to start from the left side of the wall bar and moving sideways to pass over, under and through some obstacles, following a predetermined path, without falling (Figure 1).

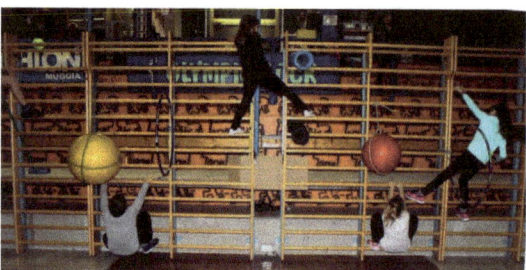

Figure 1. Children performing exercises starting from the left side of the wall bar and moving sideways to pass over.

Exercise 2: The game of spiders and crabs: half of the children have to positioning themselves in a line, keeping their arms and legs outstretched, forming a large arch. The crabs will have to come through it (Figure 2).

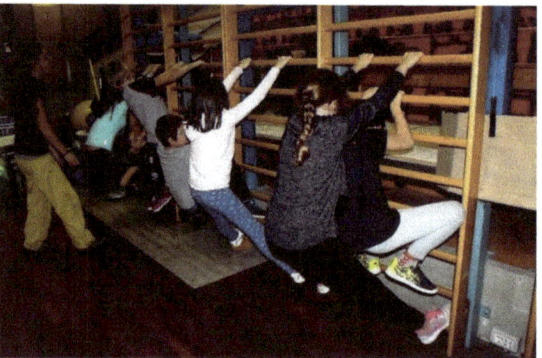

Figure 2. Overview of spider and crab positions.

The Proceritas Secunda phase: Mobilization of the spine (Figures 3 and 4a,b) and the tibio–tarsic joint (Figure 5):

Exercise 1: Hamstring stretch involving two subjects (A and B) that have to sit back-to-back on the floor with their legs extended forward. Subject A is stretching back by abducting his/her arms upwards slightly pressing its weight, and simultaneously subject B reaches for his/her toes. The position has to be kept constant for 4–5 s, after which this exercise is repeated but with the subjects changing their roles (Figure 3).

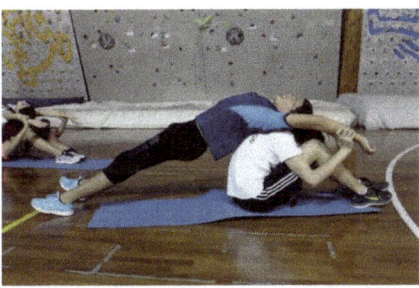

Figure 3. Final position of the spine mobilization exercise.

Exercise 2: The subjects sit up tall in the straddle position feet-to-feet, with straightened legs, and holding a ball in their hands (Figure 4a). They slowly lean down on the back, closing their legs and curling the pelvis inward until their toes touch the ball behind their heads, and then back to the starting position (Figure 4b).

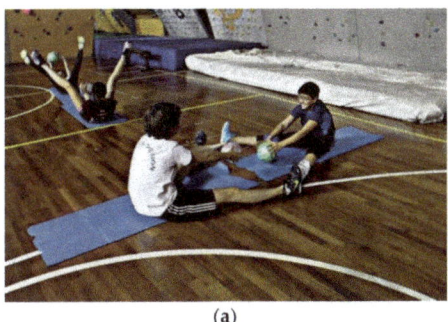 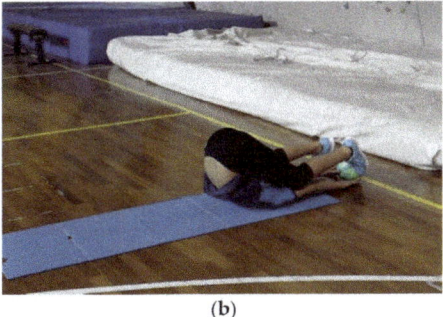

(a) (b)

Figure 4. (a) Starting position of the mobilization of the spine and coxo–femoral joint exercises. (b) Ending position of the mobilization of the spine and coxo-femoral joint exercises.

Exercise 3: In single foot support, rotate the rope forward without jumping. After rotating the rope forward, to pass the rope beyond the foot, flex the foot and then extend it. Do the same with the other foot (Figure 5).

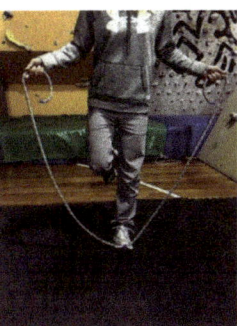

Figure 5. Flex foot and rope locked by the foot.

Turgor Tertius phase: Mobility exercises for the fingers (Figure 6), coxo–femoral (Figure 7) and tibio–tarsic joints (Figure 8):

Exercise 1: Starting with a hand fully opened; perform four closing finger movements, through which both the metacarpophalangeal and the interphalangeal joints will be stimulated (Figure 6).

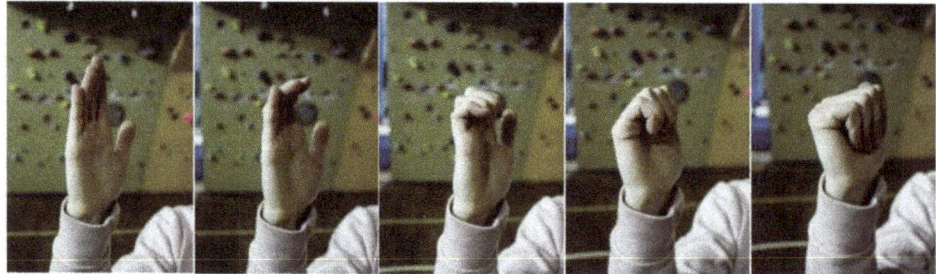

Figure 6. Mobility exercises for fingers from starting to ending positions.

Exercise 2: The subject is crouched down, the feet are in a wide stance with the toes turned out, the back outstretched, the heels on the ground and the elbows slightly pushing the knees outwards. Then, small rotations of the ankles are made first in one direction and then in the other (Figure 7).

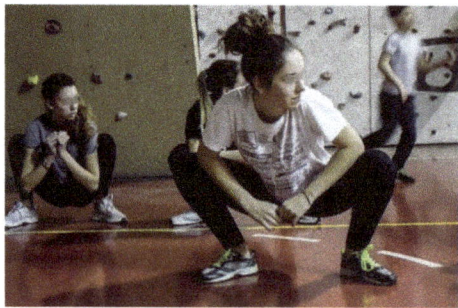

Figure 7. Squat position for mobilization of the coxo–femoral joint.

Exercise 3: Four different types of gaits are proposed. First, toe walking with raised arms. Second, heel walking with raised arms. Third, foot rolling forward. Lastly, feet supination and pronation walking forward (Figure 8A–D).

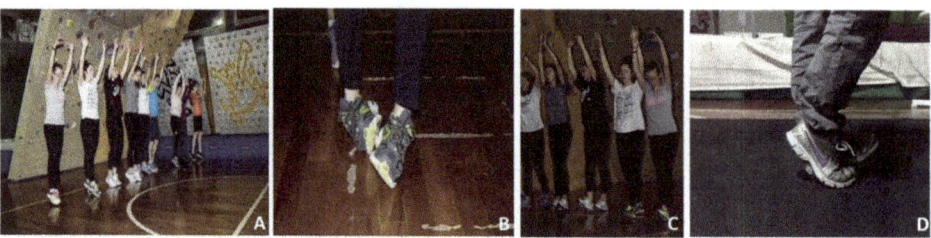

Figure 8. (**A**) Toe walking with raised arms; (**B**) foot rolling forward; (**C**) heel walking with raised arms; (**D**) feet supination and pronation walking forward.

2.4. Statistical Analysis

Data collected at baseline (pre-training) and after (post-training) the one-year experimental period are presented as the mean ± SD. The assumption of normality was verified by means of the

Kolmogorov–Smirnov test. Then, for each subgroup a paired t-student test was used to ascertain differences between pre-training and post-training data. Throughout the study, the level of significance was set at $p \leq 0.05$. Statistical analysis was conducted using GraphPad Prism version 6.

3. Results

Athletes have carried out the proposed activities for the entire duration of the study over and above the regular workout, with the exception of a female belonging to the group Proceritas Secunda who interrupted the training program for one and a half months. However, data from subjects who dropped out were used for preliminary comparisons. All groups considered in our study have shown an improvement in joint mobility (Table 2). However, differences in training response among the considered phases have been identified.

Table 2. Percentage of improvement in flexibility in the different phases expressed as mean fold change ± SD.

PHASE	SCAPULO–HUMERAL JOINT (Mean ± SD)	COXO–FEMORAL JOINT (Mean ± SD)	SPINE (Mean ± SD)
TURGOR SECUNDIS	8.19 ± 1.76	6.46 ± 0.74	35.95 ± 3.16
PROCERITAS SECUNDA	7.82 ± 1.08	8.58 ± 2.07	36.28 ± 4.15
TURGOR TERTIUS	11.85 ± 2.20	4.20 ± 1.18	27.97 ± 7.71

Proceritas Secunda showed a positive response in coxo–femoral mobility and lower vertebral column flexibility 12 months after the start of the training program (Figures 9 and 10), whereas scapula–humeral mobility did not report benefits after joint-specific training (Figure 11). On the other hand, scapula–humeral mobility remarkably improves in the Turgor Tertius phase when compared to both Turgor Secundus and Proceritas Secunda (Figure 11). Indeed, this is consistent with the normal development of the shoulder joint that tends to complement the most advanced evolutionary phases. However, this does not apply to the other two phases (Figure 11). The Turgor Tertius group have also recorded an improvement in spine flexibility as reported in Figure 10.

Regarding Proceritas Secunda, we further compared two 14-year-old subjects (Figure 12). Athlete A has completed his/her training, whereas Athlete B has totally interrupted the workout for one and a half months. The latter has been previously excluded from the overall analysis. It is noteworthy that we clearly identified a remarkable impairment in terms of mobility and flexibility as a result of the training discontinuation of Athlete B.

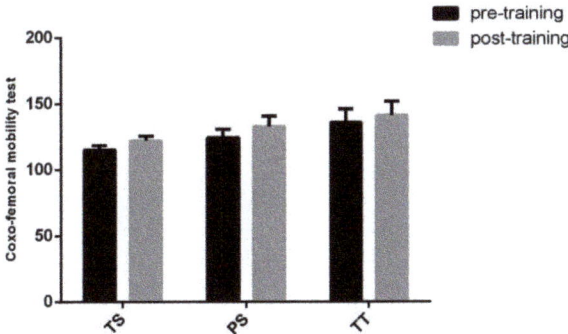

Figure 9. Coxo–femoral mobility test. The results are represented in bar graphs as the mean ± SD of the different phases considered (Turgor Secundus, Proceritas Secunda and Turgor Tertius).

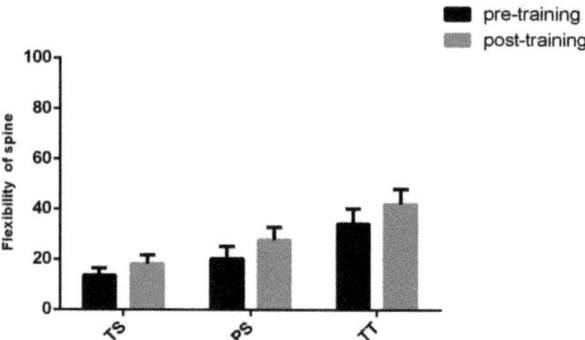

Figure 10. Flexibility of the spine. The results are represented in bar graphs as the mean ± SD of the different phases considered (Turgor Secundus, Proceritas Secunda and Turgor Tertius).

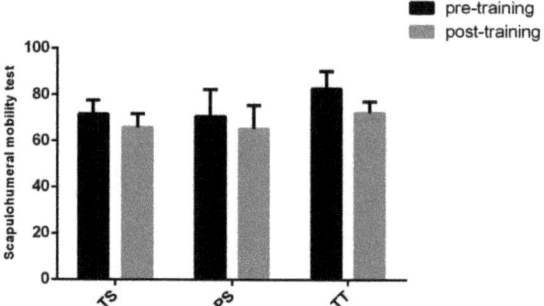

Figure 11. Scapulo–humeral mobility test. The results are represented in bar graphs as the mean ± SD of the different phases considered (Turgor Secundus, Proceritas Secunda and Turgor Tertius).

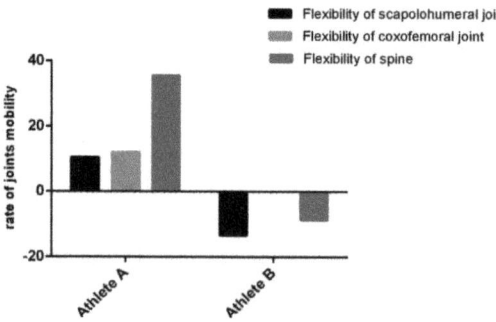

Figure 12. Comparison between the percentage mean variations of two athletes: Athlete A has completed the training, while Athlete B has totally interrupted the workout for one and a half months.

4. Discussion

This work represents a preliminary study in order to demonstrate both the efficacy on joint mobility and the requirement of our playful work, to support the global sport-climbing workout. Indeed, the increased interest in rock climbing practices creates the need to know all the possible sport-related injuries in order to prevent and treat them. Hence, the importance to study the main joints involved in climbing and that are at risk of injuries, such as joints of the hand and fingers, shoulders, the hip and ankles, in order to develop a preparation workout suitable for the discipline.

Since sport climbing does not need specific anthropometrical characteristic, and for this reason it can be practiced by everyone [30], a specific training program in this sport can improve one's strength and resistance; essential skills that would allow to carry out increasingly difficult passages. In fact, climbers perform movements that require an isometric effort, resulting in an enhanced muscle tone to obtain a strong and harmonious body. Moreover, although it is not an aerobic discipline, it develops a good cardiovascular training; this is also due to the adrenaline that develops while climbing [31].

Because of a child's incomplete maturation of both bone and muscular structures, and the laxity of ligaments, early and specific training would reasonably provide extensive room for improvement. We have proposed a playful training workout as a mobility workout in the first sensitive stages.

In the present work, we have conducted a preliminary study in an attempt to prove that a specific training program is fundamental for mobility and flexibility improvement. Participants enrolled for our study were novices regarding climbing experience and they worked out twice a week for 90 min in agreement with the coach's training plan for 12 months.

Although the reported data did not reach statistical significance, we have recorded an improvement in joint mobility after the playful training program. However, not all the recorded ameliorations were statistically significant. This might be due to external factors affecting joint mobility, such as anatomical and physiological differences among subjects. However, this can be also ascribable to the low sample size. The latter stems from the direct correlation between the standard deviation value and the sample size.

Moreover, by comparing continuous and discontinuous training between two athletes, we have suggested the importance of early and constant training (Figure 12). Indeed, the suspension of a joint-specific workout can lead to a blockage or even a regression of the subject's abilities. Thus, injuries require prompt treatment in order to avoid transient and permanent physical impairment.

Even if the study was conducted on a low number of subjects, this represent a starting project in order to develop a specific training program for each developmental phase.

5. Conclusions

The recent proliferation of indoor climbing gyms and well-protected sport climbing areas have made sport climbing accessible to everyone. Neither an age group nor a pre-existing medical condition serves as a contraindication for sport climbing in the first instance. Sport climbing is an engaging mental and physical activity that contributes to an increase in muscle mass and strength, dynamic balance, and other health benefits. However, in line with any exercise prescription, guidelines for sport-specific participation are desirable. Taking into account what was shown in this preliminary study, early and constant joint-mobility training that start from the early stages of the developmental age is fundamental.

In conclusion, we suggest that joint-mobility exercises from the early stages of development will allow children to move harmoniously, even on the climbing walls.

Author Contributions: Conceptualization, L.G. and A.G.D.; methodology, L.G.; validation, E.P. and G.A.; formal analysis, M.M. and V.T.; investigation, L.G.; data curation, A.G.D.; statistical analysis, G.M. and A.G.D.; writing—original draft preparation, M.M., A.G.D. and E.P.; writing—review and editing, M.M.; G.M. and V.T.; supervision, A.G.D. All authors read and approved the final manuscript.

Funding: This research received no external funding.

Conflicts of Interest: The authors declare no conflict of interest.

References

1. Available online: https://www.ifsc-climbing.org/index.php (accessed on 29 July 2019).
2. Available online: https://tokyo2020.org/en/ (accessed on 29 July 2019).
3. Available online: https://www.ifsc-climbing.org/ (accessed on 29 July 2019).

4. Michailov, M.L.; Baláš, J.; Tanev, S.K.; Andonov, H.S.; Kodejška, J.; Brown, L. Reliability and Validity of Finger Strength and Endurance Measurements in Rock Climbing. *Res. Q. Exerc. Sport* **2018**, *89*, 246–254. [CrossRef] [PubMed]
5. Baláš, J.; Pecha, O.; Martin, A.J.; Cochrane, D. Hand–arm strength and endurance as predictors of climbing performance. *Eur. J. Sport Sci.* **2012**, *12*, 16–25. [CrossRef]
6. Li, L.; Ru, A.; Liao, T.; Zou, S.; Niu, X.H.; Wang, Y.T. Effects of Rock Climbing Exercise on Physical Fitness among College Students: A Review Article and Meta-analysis. *Iran. J. Public Health* **2018**, *47*, 1440–1452. [CrossRef]
7. Voelcker-Rehage, C.; Godde, B.; Staudinger, U.M. Cardiovascular and Coordination Training Differentially Improve Cognitive Performance and Neural Processing in Older Adults. *Front. Hum. Neurosci.* **2011**, *5*, 1–12. [CrossRef] [PubMed]
8. Kleinstäuber, M.; Reuter, M.; Doll, N.; Fallgatter, A.J. Rock climbing and acute emotion regulation in patients with major depressive disorder in the context of a psychological inpatient treatment: A controlled pilot trial. *Psychol. Res. Behav. Manag.* **2017**, *10*, 277–281. [CrossRef] [PubMed]
9. Lutter, C.; El-Sheikh, Y.; Schöffl, I.; Schöffl, V. Sport climbing: Medical considerations for this new Olympic discipline. *Br. J. Sports Med.* **2017**, *51*, 2–3. [CrossRef] [PubMed]
10. Quaine, F.; Vigouroux, L.; Martin, L. Effect of simulated rock climbing finger postures on force sharing among the fingers. *Clin. Biomech* **2003**, *18*, 385–388. [CrossRef]
11. Roloff, I.; Schöffl, V.R.; Vigouroux, L.; Quaine, F. Biomechanical model for the determination of the forces acting on the finger pulley system. *J. Biomech.* **2006**, *39*, 915–923. [CrossRef]
12. Vigouroux, L.; Quaine, F. Fingertip force and electromyography of finger flexor muscles during a prolonged intermittent exercise in elite climbers and sedentary individuals. *J. Sports Sci.* **2006**, *24*, 181–186. [CrossRef]
13. Schöffl, V.; Einwag, F.; Strecker, W.; Schöffl, I. Strength measurement after conservatively treated pulley ruptures in climbers. *Med. Sci. Sports Exerc.* **2006**, *38*, 637–643. [CrossRef] [PubMed]
14. Schöffl, I.; Einwag, F.; Strecker, W.; Hennig, F.; Schöffl, V. Impact of taping after finger flexor tendon pulley ruptures in rock climbers. *J. Appl. Biomech.* **2007**, *23*, 52–62. [CrossRef] [PubMed]
15. Morrison, A.B.; Schöffl, V.R. Physiological responses to rock climbing in young climbers. *Br. J. Sports Med.* **2007**, *41*, 852–861. [CrossRef] [PubMed]
16. Timmons, B.W.; Leblanc, A.G.; Carson, V.; Connor Gorber, S.; Dillman, C.; Janssen, I.; Kho, M.E.; Spence, J.C.; Stearns, J.A.; Tremblay, M.S. Systematic review of physical activity and health in the early years (aged 0–4 years). *Appl. Physiol. Nutr. Metab.* **2012**, *37*, 773–792.
17. Janssen, I.; Roberts, K.C.; Thompson, W. Is adherence to the Canadian 24-Hour Movement Behaviour Guidelines for Children and Youth associated with improved indicators of physical, mental, and social health? *Appl. Physiol. Nutr. Metab.* **2017**, *42*, 725–731. [CrossRef] [PubMed]
18. Malm, C.; Jakobsson, J.; Isaksson, A. Physical Activity and Sports—Real Health Benefits: A Review with Insight into the Public Health of Sweden. *Sports* **2019**, *7*, 127. [CrossRef] [PubMed]
19. Iwame, T.; Matsuura, T.; Suzue, N.; Iwase, J.; Uemura, H.; Sairyo, K. Factors Associated With Knee Pain and Heel Pain in Youth Soccer Players Aged 8 to 12 Years. *Orthopaedic J. Sports Med.* **2019**, *7*, 2325967119883370. [CrossRef]
20. Schöffl, V.; Lutter, C.; Woollings, K.; Schöffl, I. Pediatric and adolescent injury in rock climbing. *Res. Sport. Med.* **2018**, *26*, 91–113. [CrossRef]
21. Garcia, K.; Jaramillo, D.; Rubesova, E. Ultrasound evaluation of stress injuries and physiological adaptations in the fingers of adolescent competitive rock climbers. *Pediatr. Radiol.* **2018**, *48*, 366–373. [CrossRef]
22. Roseborrough, A.; Lebec, M. Differences in static scapular position between rock climbers and a non-rock climber population. *N. Am. J. Sports Phys. Ther.* **2007**, *2*, 44–50.
23. Schöffl, V.R.; Hoffmann, P.M.; Imhoff, A.; Küpper, T.; Schöffl, I.; Hochholzer, T.; Hinterwimmer, S. Long-Term Radiographic Adaptations to Stress of High-Level and Recreational Rock Climbing in Former Adolescent Athletes: An 11-Year Prospective Longitudinal Study. *Orthop. J. Sport. Med.* **2018**, *6*, 1–9. [CrossRef]
24. Nelson, C.E.; Rayan, G.M.; Judd, D.I.; Ding, K.; Stoner, J.A. Survey of Hand and Upper Extremity Injuries Among Rock Climbers. *Hand* **2017**, *12*, 389–394. [CrossRef] [PubMed]
25. Turner, C.H.; Robling, A.G. Exercise as an anabolic stimulus for bone. *Curr. Pharm. Des.* **2004**, *10*, 2629–2641. [CrossRef]
26. Watts, P.B. Physiology of difficult rock climbing. *Eur. J. Appl. Physiol.* **2004**, *91*, 361–372. [CrossRef]

27. Anloague, P.A.; Spees, V.; Smith, J.; Herbenick, M.A.; Rubino, L.J. Glenohumeral range of motion and lower extremity flexibility in collegiate-level baseball players. *Sports Health* **2012**, *4*, 25–30. [CrossRef] [PubMed]
28. Boone, D.C.; Azen, S.P.; Lin, C.M.; Spence, C.; Baron, C.; Lee, L. Reliability of goniometric measurements. *Phys. Ther.* **1978**, *58*, 1355–1360. [CrossRef] [PubMed]
29. Sharma, J.P. *Tests and Measurements in Physical Education*; Khel Sahitya Kendra: New Delhi, Delhi, India, 2011; ISBN 8175243856.
30. Mermier, C.M.; Janot, J.M.; Parker, D.L.; Swan, J.G. Physiological and anthropometric determinants of sport climbing performance. *Br. J. Sports Med.* **2000**, *34*, 359–366. [CrossRef] [PubMed]
31. Mermier, C.M. Energy expenditure and physiological responses during indoor rock climbing. *Br. J. Sports Med.* **1997**, *31*, 224–228. [CrossRef]

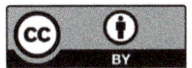

© 2020 by the authors. Licensee MDPI, Basel, Switzerland. This article is an open access article distributed under the terms and conditions of the Creative Commons Attribution (CC BY) license (http://creativecommons.org/licenses/by/4.0/).

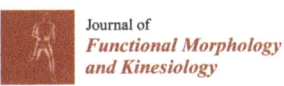

Article

Cognitive and Physical Activity-Related Aspects of Children Associated to the Performance of the Crunning Movement

Ewan Thomas [1,*], Marianna Alesi [1], Garden Tabacchi [1], Carlos Marques da Silva [2], David J. Sturm [3], Fatma Neşe Şahin [4], Özkan Güler [4], Manuel Gómez-López [5], Simona Pajaujiene [6], Michele Basile [7], Ante Rada [8], Antonio Palma [1] and Antonino Bianco [1]

1. Sport and Exercise Sciences Research Unit, Department of Psychology, Educational Science and Human Movement, University of Palermo, 90146 Palermo, Italy; marianna.alesi@unipa.it (M.A.); tabacchi.garden@libero.it (G.T.); antonio.palma@unipa.it (A.P.); antonino.bianco@unipa.it (A.B.)
2. CIEQV-Life Quality Research Centre, Escola Superior de Desporto de Rio Maior-IPSANTAREM, Avenida Dr. Mário Soares, 20413 RIO Maior, Portugal; csilva@esdrm.ipsantarem.pt
3. Department of Sport and Health Sciences, Technical University of Munich, Uptown Munich Campus D, Georg-Brauchle-Ring 60/62, 80992 Munich, Germany; david.sturm@tum.de
4. Department of Sport and Health, Faculty of Sport Sciences, Ankara University, Golbaşı Yerleşkesi Spor Bilimleri Fakültesi, Golbaşı, 06830 Ankara, Turkey; nesesahin@ankara.edu.tr (F.N.Ş.); oguler@ankara.edu.tr (Ö.G.)
5. Department of Physical Activity and Sport, Faculty of Sports Sciences, University of Murcia, Calle Argentina, s/n., 30720 Murcia, Spain; mgomezlop@um.es
6. Department of Coaching Science, Lithuanian Sports University, Sporto 6, LT-44221 Kaunas, Lithuania; simona.pajaujiene@lsu.lt
7. University of Palermo Sport Center (CUS Palermo), Via Altofonte, 80, 90129 Palermo, Italy; miter702@libero.it
8. Faculty of Kinesiology, University of Split, Teslina 6, 21000 Split, Croatia; arada@kifst.hr
* Correspondence: ewan.thomas@unipa.it; Tel.: +39-3208899934

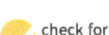

Citation: Thomas, E.; Alesi, M.; Tabacchi, G.; Silva, C.M.d.; Sturm, D.J.; Şahin, F.N.; Güler, Ö.; Gómez-López, M.; Pajaujiene, S.; Basile, M.; et al. Cognitive and Physical Activity-Related Aspects of Children Associated to the Performance of the Crunning Movement. *J. Funct. Morphol. Kinesiol.* 2021, 6, 9. https://doi.org/10.3390/jfmk6010009

Received: 16 December 2020
Accepted: 13 January 2021
Published: 17 January 2021

Publisher's Note: MDPI stays neutral with regard to jurisdictional claims in published maps and institutional affiliations.

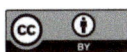

Copyright: © 2021 by the authors. Licensee MDPI, Basel, Switzerland. This article is an open access article distributed under the terms and conditions of the Creative Commons Attribution (CC BY) license (https://creativecommons.org/licenses/by/4.0/).

Abstract: The aim of this investigation was to identify possible related factors associated to the performance of the crunning test in European children and adolescents. A total number of 559 children and adolescents (age range 6–14 years) of which 308 boys (55.1%) and 251 girls (44.9%), from seven European countries, were screened. A questionnaire concerning demographic and personal life-related factors and a cognitive assessment were performed. A regression analysis was conducted with the performance measures of the crunning movement. T-tests and ANCOVA were used to analyze sub-group differences. Boys have greater crunning performance values compared to girls (5.55 s vs. 7.06 s, $p < 0.001$) and older children perform better than younger ones (R2 -0.23; $p < 0.001$). Children with healthy and active habits (exercising or spending time with family members vs. reading or surfing the internet) performed better in the test. Children engaged in team sports had better crunning performances compared to those engaged in individual sports (6.01 s vs. 6.66 s, $p = 0.0166$). No significant association was found regarding cognitive-related aspects in either children engaged in team or individual sports and the crunning performance. Older and male children performed better in the crunning test than younger and female children. Physical activity-related aspects of children's life are associated with crunning movement performance. No association was found between higher cognitive performance and the crunning test results.

Keywords: crunning; socio-demographic; cognitive; fitness-tests

1. Introduction

Physical fitness (PF) during childhood and adolescence has been deeply investigated [1–3]. It has been recognized that PF is an important health-related factor, which may predict health status in adulthood, and which may also help physical and cognitive development [1,4–6]. Inverse associations have been found between PF and cardiovascular disease, metabolic risk factors and adiposity, which overall suggest positive health-related aspects [5,7,8]. A recent review by Donnelly et al. [4], investigating the effects of PF on cognition, learning and brain structure and function in children aged 6–13 years old, found a general positive association regarding cognition and brain structure and function. However, the study failed to identify a specific set of activity parameters which may better promote the abovementioned aspects. However, despite different evidence existing regarding a positive association between physical activity (PA) and academic achievements [9], there are still inconsistencies regarding aspects of PA and cognitive function [4].

In order to promote the level of PF through PA in adulthood, it is important to adequately modify lifestyle and behaviours in childhood and adolescence [10,11]. Different investigations have suggested that children and adolescents who did not regularly practice PA are more prone to develop unhealthy habits as smoking or drinking alcohol [12,13], which would inevitably decrease PF. In addition, such aspects have also been linked to the familial socio-economic status, parental education and food habits [12,13]. Therefore, since lifestyle and familial education are important factors which influence both physical and psychological development of children and adolescence, these may be considered as important predictors of PF and health outcomes [14].

In order to quantify the levels of PF, a large body of scientific evidence exists which takes into account specific age ranges and genders [1,15–18], demographic characteristics [19–21] or more specific sub-populations [22,23]. Each investigation has evaluated different aspects related to PF, such as aerobic activity, strength, power, speed, coordination, flexibility, agility and other abilities, including for each of these, one or more field or laboratory tests to appropriately discriminate such abilities.

Despite the large number of fitness tests and physical evaluation batteries available, performance values or predictors of the crunning movement, a specific type of locomotion which combines running and crawling, are scarce. Patrick et al. [24] evaluated the inter-limb coordination during crawling in infants and adults, suggesting that a great involvement of coordination by the central nervous systems is required for quadrupedal locomotion. Other two investigations have included specific crawling exercises, within a fitness battery, to improve PF in a military environment [25,26]. The results of the studies underline that the military personnel increased the efficacy of different abilities, such as coordination, agility, speed, and power, following such interventions. Another investigation tried to determine a link between the Illinois agility test, which evaluates agility, and the crunning test. The results indicate a moderate correlation ($r = 0.45$) between the two tests [27], suggesting that a certain amount of agility is required to perform the crunning movement. In an attempt to understand if the crunning locomotion could provide further information than those offered from already known fitness tests, we included the crunning test in a previously discussed project [15]. This project, namely, the Enriched Sport Activity (ESA) program, was a physical activity intervention with the aim to improve fitness of children and adolescents across Europe by including cognitively enriched stimuli within specific warm-ups, prior to a structured physical activity [15]. However, such tests, together with the Leger shuttle run for aerobic assessment [28], were the only tests not influenced by the ESA intervention.

In order to clarify the characteristics of the crunning movement, this investigation will aim to identify lifestyle, physical activity and cognitive aspects associated with the results of this particular type of locomotion.

2. Materials and Methods

2.1. Participants

The sample was composed of 589 children of ages ranging from 6 to 14 years (aged 10.25 ± 1.76 years and 9.98 ± 1.87 years) of which 308 boys (55.1%, age 9.1 ± 1.3 years; weight, 34.9 ± 9.5 kg; height, 139.0 ± 10.4 cm) and 251 girls (44.9%, 10.2 ± 1.8 years; 39.4 ± 11.1 kg; 144.8 ± 14.3 cm), from 7 European countries (Italy, $n = 164$ of which 92 boys and 72 girls; Germany, $n = 64$ of which 41 boys and 23 girls; Portugal, $n = 111$ boys; Spain, $n = 37$ of which 17 boys and 20 girls; Lithuania, $n = 85$ of which 53 boys and 32 girls;

Croatia, n = 50 of which 25 boys and 25 girls; and Turkey, n = 78 girls) within the ESA Program, an evidence-based exercise program cofounded by the Erasmus + Program of the European Union (Key action: Sport-579661-EPP-1-2016-2-IT-SPO-SCP).

Criteria for including participants were the following: 1. Able to perform the required tests; 2. Absence of a diagnosis of intellectual disability, visual or neurological impairments; 3. Absence of a diagnosis of other neurodevelopmental disorders. All children were recruited within a school or sport center. Before the inclusion of the children in the ESA program, a parent or legal representative of each child signed a declaration of informed consent. The study was conducted in accordance with the Helsinki Declaration (Hong Kong revision, September 1989) and the European Union recommendations for Good Clinical Practice (document 111/3976/88, July 1990). The study was approved with permission from the Lithuanian Sports University's Research Ethics Committee in Social Sciences with approval No 579661-EPP-1-2016-2-IT-SPO-SCP (2018-02-05).

2.2. Study Design

The ESA Program aimed to improve children's motor skills and executive functions through sport activities enriched by cognitive stimuli to enhance inhibitory control, working memory and shifting.

Detailed description of the study design and the ESA Program can be found elsewhere, describing both the cognitive tests and their administration and motor components, as well as the full description of the crunning test and administration procedures within the project [15,29].

2.3. Intervention Procedure and Assessment Tools

Each ESA trainer underwent a training procedure before the start of the intervention, in order to adopt a standardized procedure. The procedure was shared across the participating countries. This can be also found on a dedicated YouTube channel (ESA Program). Therefore, all testing procedures were performed in the same way and order. At the beginning of the project, each participant underwent a cognitive examination [29] and a physical evaluation [15], which were repeated at the end of the intervention. Before the start of the ESA training program, each participant also underwent a psychological test battery (ESA PTB, a 32 item questionnaire which includes questions regarding personal information, lifestyle-related factors and school-associated information), which was administered on two different occasions prior to the inclusion of the participants in the ESA program. On the first day, the participants underwent a cognitive assessment which lasted around 1 h [29]. On the second day, a questionnaire was administered, which included questions related to habits, family, recreational and social aspects. We retrospectively evaluated the predicting factors of the crunning performance through these personal aspects.

The crunning performance, measured as the time in seconds needed to perform the test (10 m distance), was the dependent variable collected through the crunning test, included in the ESA fitness battery. This battery is composed of six fitness tests (standing broad jump, seated medicine ball throw, 20 m shuttle run test, 30 m sprint, Illinois test and the crunning test) to assess different skill-related components at once [30], but for the purpose of the present paper, only the outcomes of the crunning test have been considered [15]. Low values in the test measure indicate better performance.

For the purpose of this study, gender and age were treated as covariates, while a number of predictors were taken into account. These predictors included sport-related aspects, spare time-related aspects and cognitive or neuropsychological aspects.

Each aspect is discussed below.

(a) Sport-related aspects: Sport type (individual/team and exercise intensity) and sport frequency.

Individual/team sport type classification was manually distinguished by the authors on the basis of the sport practiced. The American Heart Association classification for sport was adopted [31] for grouping the activities in relation to cardiovascular function. These are divided by static and dynamic activities, and each is stratified according to exercise intensity, categorized as low, moderate or high. Current sport frequency and past sport frequency were measured in hours per week and relevant data were collected through a dedicated section of the ESA PTB.

(b) Spare time-related aspects (frequencies in h/week): Aspects regarding time spent with parents and siblings, reading, going to the cinema, theatre or museums, surfing the internet, playing with electronic games, going out with friends, going to the gym, going to the park or shopping were evaluated. All these items were collected through a dedicated section of the ESA PTB.

(c) Cognitive/neuropsychological variables: School marks (National language, Maths, Anthropology and History, Geography, Physical education, Foreign language), inhibitory control, working memory, shifting of attention. The ESA PTB was used to collect the school mark items. The other items' assessment was performed through the neuropsychological tests derived by the Inquisit Lab platform (Inquisit 6 (for Windows version 6.1). 2020. Retrieved from https://www.millisecond.com): the Color Word Stroop (CWS) task for the inhibitory control, measured by the time needed to select the right color within the stroop test; the Digit Span Test (DST) for working memory, measured by the number of recalled digits in an exact order and in a reversed order; and the Trail Making Test (TMT) for shifting of attention, measured by error number and execution time. For further details regarding the cognitive test administration, please refer to Gentile et al. [29].

2.4. Statistical Analysis

Data are presented as means and standard deviations. The Student's t-test was used to assess differences in the crunning test for each variable (i.e., gender, sport type). To estimate differences in the crunning performance by country, age range and sport type, the ANCOVA test was performed. Age and gender were used as covariates for all analysis.

Linear regression analyses were performed to evaluate correlations between the crunning test and sport frequency, spare time-related aspects, cognitive/neuropsychological aspects. Statistical significance was set for $p < 0.05$. All estimates were adjusted for gender and age. The software STATA/MP 12.1 (StataCorp. 2011. Stata Statistical Software: Release 12. College Station, TX, USA: StataCorp LP.) was used for the statistical analysis.

3. Results

3.1. Gender and Age

Mean time to perform the crunning test was 6.25 s (SD 2.416, $n.$ = 589). Better crunning performances were observed for males compared to females (independently from age) and for older compared to younger children (independently from gender) (Table 1). The regression coefficient for age was -0.23 (SE 0.051, $p = 0.000$, $n = 589$).

Table 1. Differences in the crunning test performances by gender and age range.

	n	Mean (s)	SD (s)	p-Value
Tot	589	6.25	2.416	
Gender				0.000 [a]
male	318	5.55	2.306	
female	271	7.06	2.289	
Age range				0.000 [b]
6–8	162	7.2	2.946	
9–11	298	5.99	1.97	
≥12	129	5.65	2.291	

SD: Standard deviation; Tot: Total number; [a] Estimated through paired Student's t-test. [b] Estimated through ANCOVA. All estimates were adjusted for gender and age.

3.2. Demographic Factors

Table 2 shows the differences in the crunning movement performances by demographic and SES factors. Similar characteristics across participants for each county were observed (Italy, 8.5 ± 1 years; 34.3 ± 9.8 kg; 135.0 ± 9.8 cm; boys, 8.4 ± 1 years; 33.9 ± 9.7 kg; 135.3 ± 9.7 cm and girls, 8.6 ± 1.1 years; 34.8 ± 10.1 kg; 134.7 ± 10 cm; Germany, 8.9 ± 0.8 years; 37.6 ± 9.9 kg; 137.8 ± 7.5 cm; boys, 9.0 ± 0.8 years; 37.6 ± 8.4 kg; 138.6 ± 7.3 cm and girls, 8.7 ± 0.7 years; 37.4 ± 12.7 kg; 136.3 ± 7.9 cm; Portugal, boys, 10.9 ± 1.7 years; 139.1 ± 15.3 cm; 39.4 ± 9.3 kg; Spain, 10.5 ± 1.0 years; 142.7 ± 20.4 cm; 45.1 ± 23.1 kg; boys, 10.4 ± 0.9 years; 145.8 ± 14.1 cm; 43.2 ± 12.4 kg and girls, 10.4 ± 1.0 years; 144.7 ± 13.2 cm; 40.2 ± 10.4 kg; Lithuania, 9.9 ± 1.13 years; 35.7 ± 8.0 kg; 144.0 ± 9.0 cm, boys 9.9 ± 1.19 years; 36.4 ± 8.9 kg; 144.0 ± 9.0 cm and girls 10.1 ± 1.02 years; 34.6 ± 5.8 kg; 142.0 ± 11.0 cm; Croatia 9.4 ± 0.5 years; 35.0 ± 8.2 kg; 138.3 ± 7.6 cm; boys, 9.7 ± 0.5 years; 36.5 ± 7.6 kg; 140.7 ± 7.4 cm and girls, 9.3 ± 0.5 years; 34.7 ± 8.3 kg; 137.8 ± 7.6 cm; and Turkey, girls, 10.8 ± 1.8 years; 134.9 ± 12.7 cm; 45.3 ± 10.9 kg). Significant differences in the crunning movement were found across countries.

Table 2. Differences in crunning test performances by country and socio-economic status.

	n	Mean (s)	SD (s)	p-Value [a]
Country	589	6.25	2.416	0.000
Croatia	50	5.26	1.325	
Germany	64	5.62	3.116	
Italy	164	7.69	2.501	
Lithuania	85	5.36	1.503	
Portugal	111	4.31	1.151	
Spain	37	6.37	0.508	
Turkey	78	8.03	1.709	

SD: Standard deviation; [a] Estimated through ANCOVA. All estimates were adjusted for gender and age.

3.3. Sport-Related Aspects

Among the sport-related aspects, the following were found to be associated to better performances: team sport type, with children practicing team sports performing better than those practicing individual sports (h/week) (Table 3).

Table 3. Differences in crunning test performances by sport-related aspects.

	n	Mean (s)	SD (s)	p-Value [a]
Sport type	384	6.18	2.316	0.0166
Individual	104	6.64	2.321	
Team	280	6.01	2.294	
Sport type (n = 5 *)	384	6.18	2.316	0.1139
	n.	R^2.	SE	p-value [b]
Sport frequency (h/week)	467	0.14	0.101	0.168

SD: Standard deviation; SE: Standard error; [a] Estimated through paired Student's t-test. [b] Estimated through linear regression analysis. * Five sport categories were included, according to the American Heart Association classification adopted.

No differences were found across different sports, current sport frequency, sport type (based on the American Heart Association classification (impact)).

3.4. Spare Time-Related Aspects

Regarding spare time-related aspects, the following items were correlated to the crunning performances. In general, physical activities such as attending a gym, going to the park or going out with friends were positively associated to performance outcomes (Table 4).

Table 4. Differences in crunning test performances by spare time-related aspects. All estimates were adjusted for gender and age.

Activity (Times/Week)	n	R^2	SE	p-Value [a]
Going to the gym	531	−0.16	0.079	0.049
Going to the park	537	−0.29	0.094	0.002
Going out with friends	534	−0.25	0.078	0.002
Shopping	538	−0.06	0.097	0.53
Going to the cinema/theatre/museum	532	−0.1	0.128	0.447
Surfing the internet	538	−0.06	0.071	0.417
Playing electronic games	538	0.13	0.07	0.056
Reading	539	−0.05	0.075	0.535
Spending more time with parents and siblings	541	−0.17	0.087	0.049

SE: Standard error; [a] Estimated through linear regression analysis. All estimates were adjusted for gender and age.

Furthermore, spending more time with parents and siblings seems to be associated with better performances.

3.5. Cognitive/Neuropsychological Aspects

In general, very low regression coefficients were found. Children with lower school marks had better crunning performances, such relation was present in either children practicing teams and individual sports (Table 5). No significant correlations were found between all the inhibitory control items and the crunning movement for children practicing team or individual sports, with higher times needed to select congruent, incongruent and control trials associated to lower times needed to perform the test. Working memory items were not correlated to the crunning performance.

Table 5. Associations between the crunning test performance and cognitive/neuropsychological aspects for team and individual sport practitioners.

	Team				Individual			
	n	$R^{2\,a}$	SE	p	n	$R^{2\,a}$	SE	p
School marks								
National language	205	0.47	1.58	0.000	75	0.15	0.40	0.012
Maths	70	0.29	2.49	0.000	77	0.15	0.33	0.009
Anthropology and History	65	0.19	2.49	0.000	73	0.11	0.31	0.041
Physical Activity	62	0.22	2.44	0.003	76	0.17	0.51	0.004
Foreign language	66	0.28	2.27	0.000	68	0.14	0.37	0.027
Inhibitory control (CWS)								
Congruent trial selection (s)	150	−0.59	9.03	0.845	91	−0.39	2.15	0.735
Incongruent trial selection (s)	150	0.69	2.17	0.182	91	0.55	2.21	0.116
Control trial selection (s)	150	0.39	2.18	0.004	91	0.50	2.59	0.254
Working memory (DST)								
Forward recall of numbers (n)	156	0.16	0.89	0.000	77	0.07	0.55	0.064
Forward recall of numbers before 2 consecutive errors (n)	156	0.20	1.38	0.000	77	0.08	0.55	0.060
Backward recall of numbers (n)	156	0.15	0.129	0.000	77	0.12	0.52	0.017
Backward recall of numbers before 2 consecutive errors (n)	156	0.15	1.19	0.000	77	0.06	0.53	0.126
Shifting of attention (TMT)								
Errors in numbers (n)	148	0.18	1.05	0.000	79	0.06	0.44	0.138
Time in numbers (s)	148	0.00	0.000	0.018	79	0.00	0.000	0.256
Errors in numbers and letters (n)	148	0.23	1.26	0.000	79	0.18	0.32	0.024
Time in numbers and letters (s)	148	−0.00	0.000	0.000	79	−0.00	0.000	0.118

SE: Standard error; [a] Estimated through linear regression analysis. All estimates were adjusted for gender and age.

Items related to the shifting of attention showed positive but very low correlations to crunning times (with higher number of errors and higher time to perform the test correlated to lower crunning performances), with the only exception of the time to recognize numbers and letters in children engaged in team sports, which revealed significant correlation but very low coefficients.

4. Discussion

With this investigation, we aimed to determine possible factors associated with the performance of the crunning movement. As expected, in our population of European children, males performed better compared to females and older children performed better than younger ones.

Such aspects have been reported by various authors across different motor domains. Tomkinson et al. [1] reported for a sample of over 2 million children performances, increases across age groups from 9 to 17 years old, with males performing better than females in terms of strength, power, agility and aerobic capacity. However, the results are in favour of females regarding balance, flexibility and coordination. Similar results are reported by another investigation in a sample of 3804 children ranging between 6 to 10 years of age. Again, boys perform better than girls regarding strength, power, speed, agility and aerobic capacity but not flexibility, with performance increases according to age [32]. Both aspects are consistent with growth and physical maturation [33,34].

4.1. Demographic Aspects

The results we obtained regarding the crunning movement performance show differences related to each country with better performances from the Portuguese children and worst performances from the Turkish children. It has to be noted that the Portuguese sample was composed only of male children, while the Turkish sample was composed only of female children. Such results are consistent with the general outcomes provided above. Furthermore, it is not uncommon to appreciate geographical differences when considering different populations of same age ranges, for example, regarding speed in the 20 m sprint between 6-year-old Greek (5.05 ± 1 s) [35] and Lithuanian boys (5.8 ± 1.2 s) [36], or for jumping performance of 10-year-old Colombian girls [20] (110.2 cm), Australian girls (103.25 cm) [37] or South African girls (149.3 cm) [38] in the standing long jump. Differences are also present between the same country when considering rural and city areas [39]. The authors of this latter study indicated that these differences between areas possibly influence individual habits and therefore the level of physical activity which each children experiences. A review by Carlin et al. [40] also analysed the association of environmental factors and levels of PA. The study associated increased levels of PA in neighbourhoods which provided facilities, parks and public equipment, and found the opposite for those with fewer facilities. Therefore, environmental and cultural aspects may possibly explain the difference reported between the test performance of each country within the present investigation.

4.2. Sport and Spare Time-Related Aspects

In the previous sections, the influence of habits regarding the activity levels was evaluated [41]. The results we obtained in this sample of European children confirm that positive habits and lifestyles are associated with improved performance of the crunning movement. For instance, the better results obtained in those children engaged in gym activities or those going out to the park in their spare time. Our results are in line with a systematic review analysing the relationship between outdoor time and PF in children [42]. The authors report an overall positive effect of outdoor time on PF, however, with no specific effect on musculoskeletal fitness. Another cross-sectional investigation aimed to understand how sedentary behaviours or screen time could affect motor skills in children aged 5–16 years [43]. Screen time in particular was associated with lower physical activity, with greater effects on adolescents compared to children and on girls compared to boys.

This aspect, if linked to increased sedentary behaviours, could lead to increased fat mass and therefore decreased PF amongst children [44].

In addition, our results also show that children engaged in team sports performed better than those engaged in individual activities, independently of the activity intensity. Other investigations comparing individual and team sports have reported similar results, for example, Morano et al. [45] evaluated physical and psychological factors among children, finding that children engaged in team activities had better shuttle run results for aerobic performances compared to their peers who were engaged in individual sports, and were also less dissatisfied with their body image. Jukic et al. [46] examined the differences in fundamental motor skills in a sample of under-10 soccer players, indicating that greater motor skills were positively related to gross motor quotient and locomotion skills. School children's enjoyment and cohesion during sport activities can predict physical improvements, and those engaged in team sports show significantly higher levels of enjoyment [47]. Being engaged in team sports has also been associated in children with increased motor skill proficiency [48], with greater associations in boys compared to girls. When neurobiological integrations are analysed, it is possible to see that boys involved in team sports have thinner cortices in the frontal lobe compared to those engaged in individual activities. This aspect indicates a faster maturation of the frontal cortex related to an advantage of frontal areas functioning [49]. These are factors that altogether are determinant to adequately perform a complex skill as the crunning movement, which requires the use of upper and lower limbs simultaneously.

4.3. Cognitive and Neuropsychological Aspects

Relative to cognitive and neuropsychological aspects, two main findings have been associated to the performance. Firstly, academic achievement is negatively linked to the performance results and, secondly, cognitive function is not linked to crunning performance neither for children practicing team sports nor for those practicing individual sports. Our findings are generally in contrast with other investigations. Emerging literature has positively linked cognitive performance and academic achievement to sport performance [50]. Such associations are also seen in intervention studies where both cognitive functioning and academic achievement are increased following a physical intervention [51–53]. However, the majority of studies have proposed aerobic activity as the main typology of physical activity included within their interventions [54]. These interventions are seen to act by improving brain structure and function [4]. However, within our study, neither a longitudinal intervention was undertaken nor the crunning movement involves aerobic metabolism activation. It is possible that the nature of the crunning movement itself requires a different cognitive demand compared to the cognitive and neuropsychological measures assessed.

Limitations of this study are the following: (1) The sample for each country was collected within one school, therefore, it was not possible to evaluate specific local aspects but only broad geographical differences. (2) Not all countries had the availability of both male and female participants. (3) The classification for sport intensity was based on broad characteristics of sporting activities (i.e., soccer, basket, gymnastics, etc.), therefore it is not possible to associate specific aspects related to different approaches between countries. (4) Regarding the cognitive and neuropsychological assessment, not all children and adolescents from the different countries were screened because they were not present at the time of the evaluation. Therefore, the sample which is available for providing information regarding results for such aspects is restricted. Indeed, a broader sample would be required for greater consistency of the test. There is a need to identify the sensitivity of the test to specific physical qualities.

Therefore, it will be important in future investigations to compare the present results to other populations in order to verify the applicability of the findings here provided.

The present study is the first known study to have evaluated and tried to identify variables associated to the crunning movement. Therefore, it will be necessary to consider gender and physical activity differences among individuals if planning to include the crunning test within a test battery.

5. Conclusions

The present investigation detected different factors associated with the performance of the crunning movement. These are related to lifestyle and cognitive factors which may influence performance of the crunning movement. These associated variables need to be considered when comparing the results of the crunning movement test, especially across populations. Special attention must be paid regarding gender and previously practiced physical activity. The specificity of the crunning test still needs to be understood within the context of a fitness evaluation.

Author Contributions: Conceptualization, A.B.; Data curation, A.B. and F.N.Ş.; Formal analysis, E.T. and G.T.; Investigation, C.M.d.S., M.B., M.G.-L. and S.P.; Methodology, M.G.-L.; Project administration, M.A. and A.P.; Supervision, M.B.; Visualization, A.R.; Writing—original draft, E.T. and G.T.; Writing—review & editing, A.B., Ö.G. and D.J.S. All authors have read and agreed to the published version of the manuscript.

Funding: The work was conducted within the ESA (Enriched Sport Activities) Program—Agreement number 2016-3723/001-001, funded by the Erasmus Plus Sport Programme (2017–2019) of the European Commission. Erasmus+ Sport Programme. EAC/A04/2015—Round 2 E+ SPORT PROJECT: 579661-EPP-1-2016-2-IT-SPO-SCP. Enriched Sport Activities Program.

Institutional Review Board Statement: The study was conducted according to the guidelines of the Declaration of Helsinki, and approved by the Lithuanian Sports University's Institutional Review Board, approval No 579661-EPP-1-2016-2-IT-SPO-SCP (2018-02-05).

Informed Consent Statement: A parent or legal representative of each child signed a declaration of informed consent.

Data Availability Statement: Data available on request due to restrictions eg privacy or ethical.

Conflicts of Interest: The authors declare no conflict of interest. The funders had no role in the design of the study; in the collection, analyses, or interpretation of data; in the writing of the manuscript, or in the decision to publish the results.

References

1. Tomkinson, G.R.; Carver, K.D.; Atkinson, F.; Daniell, N.D.; Lewis, L.K.; Fitzgerald, J.S.; Lang, J.J.; Ortega, F.B. European normative values for physical fitness in children and adolescents aged 9-17 years: Results from 2,779,165 eurofit performances representing 30 countries. *Br. J. Sports Med.* **2017**, *52*. [CrossRef] [PubMed]
2. Bianco, A.; Jemni, M.; Thomas, E.; Patti, A.; Paoli, A.; Ramos Roque, J.; Palma, A.; Mammina, C.; Tabacchi, G. A systematic review to determine reliability and usefulness of the field-based test batteries for the assessment of physical fitness in adolescents—The asso project. *Int. J. Occup. Med. Environ. Health* **2015**, *28*, 445–478. [CrossRef] [PubMed]
3. Ortega, F.B.; Ruiz, J.R.; Castillo, M.J.; Moreno, L.A.; Gonzalez-Gross, M.; Warnberg, J.; Gutierrez, A.; Group, A. Low level of physical fitness in spanish adolescents. Relevance for future cardiovascular health (avena study). *Rev. Esp. Cardiol.* **2005**, *58*, 898–909. [CrossRef] [PubMed]
4. Donnelly, J.E.; Hillman, C.H.; Castelli, D.; Etnier, J.L.; Lee, S.; Tomporowski, P.; Lambourne, K.; Szabo-Reed, A.N. Physical activity, fitness, cognitive function, and academic achievement in children: A systematic review. *Med. Sci. Sports Exerc.* **2016**, *48*, 1197–1222. [CrossRef]
5. Smith, J.J.; Eather, N.; Morgan, P.J.; Plotnikoff, R.C.; Faigenbaum, A.D.; Lubans, D.R. The health benefits of muscular fitness for children and adolescents: A systematic review and meta-analysis. *Sports Med.* **2014**, *44*, 1209–1223. [CrossRef]
6. Misuraca, R.; Miceli, S.; Teuscher, U. Three effective ways to nurture our brain: Physical activity, healthy nutrition, and music. A review. *Eur. Psychol.* **2017**, *22*, 101–120. [CrossRef]
7. Seo, Y.G.; Lim, H.; Kim, Y.; Ju, Y.S.; Lee, H.J.; Jang, H.B.; Park, S.I.; Park, K.H. The effect of a multidisciplinary lifestyle intervention on obesity status, body composition, physical fitness, and cardiometabolic risk markers in children and adolescents with obesity. *Nutrients* **2019**, *11*, 137. [CrossRef]
8. Karatoprak, C.; Ekinci, I.; Batar, N.; Zorlu, M.; Cakirca, M.; Kiskac, M.; Demirtunc, R. The relationship between the frequency of brisk walking and weight loss and other metabolic parameters in obese individuals. *Acta Med. Mediterr.* **2019**, 2125. [CrossRef]
9. Álvarez-Bueno, C.; Pesce, C.; Cavero-Redondo, I.; Sánchez-López, M.; Garrido-Miguel, M.; Martínez-Vizcaíno, V. Academic achievement and physical activity: A meta-analysis. *Pediatrics* **2017**, *140*, e20171498. [CrossRef]

10. Slawta, J.; Bentley, J.; Smith, J.; Kelly, J.; Syman-Degler, L. Promoting healthy lifestyles in children: A pilot program of be a fit kid. *Health Promot. Pract.* **2008**, *9*, 305–312. [CrossRef]
11. Condello, G.; Puggina, A.; Aleksovska, K.; Buck, C.; Burns, C.; Cardon, G.; Carlin, A.; Simon, C.; Ciarapica, D.; Coppinger, T.; et al. Behavioral determinants of physical activity across the life course: A "determinants of diet and physical activity" (dedipac) umbrella systematic literature review. *Int. J. Behav. Nutr. Phys. Act.* **2017**, *14*, 58. [CrossRef] [PubMed]
12. Tabacchi, G.; Faigenbaum, A.; Jemni, M.; Thomas, E.; Capranica, L.; Palma, A.; Breda, J.; Bianco, A. Profiles of physical fitness risk behaviours in school adolescents from the asso project: A latent class analysis. *Int. J. Environ. Res. Public Health* **2018**, *15*, 1933. [CrossRef] [PubMed]
13. Zaqout, M.; Vyncke, K.; Moreno, L.A.; De Miguel-Etayo, P.; Lauria, F.; Molnar, D.; Lissner, L.; Hunsberger, M.; Veidebaum, T.; Tornaritis, M.; et al. Determinant factors of physical fitness in european children. *Int. J. Public Health* **2016**, *61*, 573–582. [CrossRef] [PubMed]
14. Chung, J.W.; Chung, L.M.; Chen, B. The impact of lifestyle on the physical fitness of primary school children. *J. Clin. Nurs.* **2009**, *18*, 1002–1009. [CrossRef]
15. Thomas, E.; Bianco, A.; Tabacchi, G.; Marques da Silva, C.; Loureiro, N.; Basile, M.; Giaccone, M.; Sturm, D.J.; Sahin, F.N.; Guler, O.; et al. Effects of a physical activity intervention on physical fitness of schoolchildren: The enriched sport activity program. *Int. J. Environ. Res. Public Health* **2020**, *17*, 1723. [CrossRef]
16. Thomas, E.; Palma, A. Physical fitness evaluation of school children in southern italy: A cross sectional evaluation. *J. Funct. Morphol. Kinesiol.* **2018**, *3*, 14. [CrossRef]
17. De Miguel-Etayo, P.; Gracia-Marco, L.; Ortega, F.B.; Intemann, T.; Foraita, R.; Lissner, L.; Oja, L.; Barba, G.; Michels, N.; Tornaritis, M.; et al. Physical fitness reference standards in european children: The idefics study. *Int. J. Obes.* **2014**, *38* (Suppl. S2), S57–S66. [CrossRef]
18. Thomas, E.; Petrigna, L.; Tabacchi, G.; Teixeira, E.; Pajaujiene, S.; Sturm, D.J.; Nese Sahin, F.; Gómez-López, M.; Pausic, J.; Paoli, A.; et al. Percentile values of the standing broad jump in children and adolescents aged 6-18 years old. *Eur. J. Transl. Myol.* **2020**, *30*, 240–246. [CrossRef]
19. Hoffmann, M.D.; Colley, R.C.; Doyon, C.Y.; Wong, S.L.; Tomkinson, G.R.; Lang, J.J. Normative-referenced percentile values for physical fitness among canadians. *Health Rep.* **2019**, *30*, 14–22.
20. Ramos-Sepúlveda, J.A.; Ramírez-Vélez, R.; Correa-Bautista, J.E.; Izquierdo, M.; García-Hermoso, A. Physical fitness and anthropometric normative values among colombian-indian schoolchildren. *BMC Public Health* **2016**, *16*, 962. [CrossRef]
21. Vanhelst, J.; Labreuche, J.; Béghin, L.; Drumez, E.; Fardy, P.S.; Chapelot, D.; Mikulovic, J.; Ulmer, Z. Physical fitness reference standards in french youth: The bouge program. *J. Strength Cond. Res.* **2017**, *31*, 1709–1718. [CrossRef] [PubMed]
22. Gahche, J.J.; Kit, B.K.; Fulton, J.E.; Carroll, D.D.; Rowland, T. Normative values for cardiorespiratory fitness testing among us children aged 6-11 years. *Pediatr. Exerc. Sci.* **2017**, *29*, 177–185. [CrossRef] [PubMed]
23. Laurson, K.R.; Saint-Maurice, P.F.; Welk, G.J.; Eisenmann, J.C. Reference curves for field tests of musculoskeletal fitness in u.s. Children and adolescents: The 2012 nhanes national youth fitness survey. *J. Strength Cond. Res.* **2017**, *31*, 2075–2082. [CrossRef] [PubMed]
24. Patrick, S.K.; Noah, J.A.; Yang, J.F. Interlimb coordination in human crawling reveals similarities in development and neural control with quadrupeds. *J. Neurophysiol.* **2009**, *101*, 603–613. [CrossRef]
25. Sporiš, G.; Harasin, D.; Bok, D.; Matika, D.; Vuleta, D. Effects of a training program for special operations battalion on soldiers' fitness characteristics. *J. Strength Cond. Res.* **2012**, *26*, 2872–2882. [CrossRef]
26. Jetté, M.; Kimick, A.; Sidney, K. Evaluating the occupational physical fitness of canadian forces infantry personnel. *Mil. Med.* **1989**, *154*, 318–322. [CrossRef]
27. Feka, K.; Bianco, A. Illinois test vs crunning test in children living in southern italy: An update of the esa program. In Proceedings of the XI Congresso Nazionale SISMES, Bologna, Italy, 27–29 September 2019.
28. Leger, L.A.; Mercier, D.; Gadoury, C.; Lambert, J. The multistage 20 metre shuttle run test for aerobic fitness. *J. Sports Sci.* **1988**, *6*, 93–101. [CrossRef]
29. Gentile, A.; Boca, S.; Şahin, F.N.; Güler, Ö.; Pajaujiene, S.; Indriuniene, V.; Demetriou, Y.; Sturm, D.; Gómez-López, M.; Bianco, A.; et al. The effect of an enriched sport program on children's executive functions: The esa program. *Front. Psychol.* **2020**, *11*, 657. [CrossRef]
30. Tabacchi, G.; Lopez Sanchez, G.F.; Nese Sahin, F.; Kizilyalli, M.; Genchi, R.; Basile, M.; Kirkar, M.; Silva, C.; Loureiro, N.; Teixeira, E.; et al. Field-based tests for the assessment of physical fitness in children and adolescents practicing sport: A systematic review within the esa program. *Sustainability* **2019**, *11*, 7187. [CrossRef]
31. Levine, B.D.; Baggish, A.L.; Kovacs, R.J.; Link, M.S.; Maron, M.S.; Mitchell, J.H. Eligibility and disqualification recommendations for competitive athletes with cardiovascular abnormalities: Task force 1: Classification of sports: Dynamic, static, and impact: A scientific statement from the american heart association and american college of cardiology. *J. Am. Coll. Cardiol.* **2015**, *66*, 2350–2355.
32. Roriz De Oliveira, M.S.; Seabra, A.; Freitas, D.; Eisenmann, J.C.; Maia, J. Physical fitness percentile charts for children aged 6–10 from portugal. *J. Sports Med. Phys. Fit.* **2014**, *54*, 780–792.

33. Castro-Pinero, J.; Gonzalez-Montesinos, J.L.; Mora, J.; Keating, X.D.; Girela-Rejon, M.J.; Sjostrom, M.; Ruiz, J.R. Percentile values for muscular strength field tests in children aged 6 to 17 years: Influence of weight status. *J. Strength Cond. Res.* **2009**, *23*, 2295–2310. [CrossRef] [PubMed]
34. Marini, M.; Veicsteinas, A. The exercised skeletal muscle: A review. *Eur. J. Transl. Myol.-Myol. Rev.* **2013**, *20*, 105–120. [CrossRef]
35. Koulouvaris, P.; Tsolakis, C.; Tsekouras, Y.E.; Donti, O.; Papagelopoulos, P.J. Obesity and physical fitness indices of children aged 5-12 years living on remote and isolated islands. *Rural Remote Health* **2018**, *18*, 4425. [CrossRef]
36. Emeljanovas, A.; Mieziene, B.; Cesnaitiene, V.J.; Fjortoft, I.; Kjønniksen, L. Physical fitness and anthropometric values among lithuanian primary school children: Population-based cross-sectional study. *J. Strength Cond. Res.* **2020**, *34*, 414–421. [CrossRef] [PubMed]
37. Cochrane, T.; Davey, R.C.; de Castella, F.R. Anthropometric standards for australian primary school children: Towards a system for monitoring and supporting children's development. *J. Sci. Med. Sport* **2017**, *20*, 284–289. [CrossRef] [PubMed]
38. Armstrong, M.E.; Lambert, E.V.; Lambert, M.I. Physical fitness of south african primary school children, 6 to 13 years of age: Discovery vitality health of the nation study. *Percept. Mot. Skills* **2011**, *113*, 999–1016. [CrossRef] [PubMed]
39. Tinazci, C.; Emiroglu, O. Physical fitness of rural children compared with urban children in north cyprus: A normative study. *J. Phys. Act. Health* **2009**, *6*, 88–92. [CrossRef]
40. Carlin, A.; Perchoux, C.; Puggina, A.; Aleksovska, K.; Buck, C.; Burns, C.; Cardon, G.; Chantal, S.; Ciarapica, D.; Condello, G.; et al. A life course examination of the physical environmental determinants of physical activity behaviour: A "determinants of diet and physical activity" (dedipac) umbrella systematic literature review. *PLoS ONE* **2017**, *12*, e0182083. [CrossRef]
41. Di Maio, G.; Monda, V.; Messina, A.; Polito, R.; Monda, M.; Tartaglia, N.; Ambrosio, A.; Pisanelli, D.; Asmundo, A.; Di Nunno, N.; et al. Physical activity and modification of lifestyle induce benefits on the health status. *Acta Med. Mediterr.* **2020**, *36*, 1913–1919.
42. Gray, C.; Gibbons, R.; Larouche, R.; Sandseter, E.B.; Bienenstock, A.; Brussoni, M.; Chabot, G.; Herrington, S.; Janssen, I.; Pickett, W.; et al. What is the relationship between outdoor time and physical activity, sedentary behaviour, and physical fitness in children? A systematic review. *Int. J. Environ. Res. Public Health* **2015**, *12*, 6455–6474. [CrossRef] [PubMed]
43. Hardy, L.L.; Ding, D.; Peralta, L.R.; Mihrshahi, S.; Merom, D. Association between sitting, screen time, fitness domains, and fundamental motor skills in children aged 5-16 years: Cross-sectional population study. *J. Phys. Act. Health* **2018**, *15*, 933–940. [CrossRef] [PubMed]
44. Carson, V.; Hunter, S.; Kuzik, N.; Gray, C.E.; Poitras, V.J.; Chaput, J.P.; Saunders, T.J.; Katzmarzyk, P.T.; Okely, A.D.; Connor Gorber, S.; et al. Systematic review of sedentary behaviour and health indicators in school-aged children and youth: An update. *Appl. Physiol. Nutr. Metab.* **2016**, *41*, S240–S265. [CrossRef] [PubMed]
45. Morano, M.; Colella, D.; Capranica, L. Body image, perceived and actual physical abilities in normal-weight and overweight boys involved in individual and team sports. *J. Sports Sci.* **2011**, *29*, 355–362. [CrossRef]
46. Jukic, I.; Prnjak, K.; Zoellner, A.; Tufano, J.J.; Sekulic, D.; Salaj, S. The importance of fundamental motor skills in identifying differences in performance levels of u10 soccer players. *Sports* **2019**, *7*, 178. [CrossRef]
47. Elbe, A.M.; Wikman, J.M.; Zheng, M.; Larsen, M.N.; Nielsen, G.; Krustrup, P. The importance of cohesion and enjoyment for the fitness improvement of 8-10-year-old children participating in a team and individual sport school-based physical activity intervention. *Eur. J. Sport Sci.* **2017**, *17*, 343–350. [CrossRef]
48. Field, S.; Temple, V. The relationship between fundamental motor skill proficiency and participation in organized sports and active recreation in middle childhood. *Sports* **2017**, *5*, 43. [CrossRef]
49. Lopez-Vicente, M.; Tiemeier, H.; Wildeboer, A.; Muetzel, R.L.; Verhulst, F.C.; Jaddoe, V.W.V.; Sunyer, J.; White, T. Cortical structures associated with sports participation in children: A population-based study. *Dev. Neuropsychol.* **2017**, *42*, 58–69. [CrossRef]
50. de Greeff, J.W.; Bosker, R.J.; Oosterlaan, J.; Visscher, C.; Hartman, E. Effects of physical activity on executive functions, attention and academic performance in preadolescent children: A meta-analysis. *J. Sci. Med. Sport* **2018**, *21*, 501–507. [CrossRef]
51. Memarmoghaddam, M.; Torbati, H.T.; Sohrabi, M.; Mashhadi, A.; Kashi, A. Effects of a selected exercise programon executive function of children with attention deficit hyperactivity disorder. *J. Med. Life* **2016**, *9*, 373–379.
52. Donnelly, J.E.; Hillman, C.H.; Greene, J.L.; Hansen, D.M.; Gibson, C.A.; Sullivan, D.K.; Poggio, J.; Mayo, M.S.; Lambourne, K.; Szabo-Reed, A.N.; et al. Physical activity and academic achievement across the curriculum: Results from a 3-year cluster-randomized trial. *Prev. Med.* **2017**, *99*, 140–145. [CrossRef] [PubMed]
53. Cascone, C.; Nicotra, R.; Mangano, T.; Massimino, S.; Maugeri, A.; Petralia, M.; Attinà, A.N. Executive functions and sport climbing in adolescence. *Acta Med. Mediterr.* **2013**, *29*, 91–94.
54. Verburgh, L.; Königs, M.; Scherder, E.J.A.; Oosterlaan, J. Physical exercise and executive functions in preadolescent children, adolescents and young adults: A meta-analysis. *Br. J. Sports Med.* **2014**, *48*, 973. [CrossRef] [PubMed]

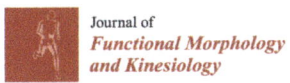

Article

Four Minutes of Sprint Interval Training Had No Acute Effect on Improving Alertness, Mood, and Memory of Female Primary School Children and Secondary School Adolescents: A Randomized Controlled Trial

Terence Chua [1], Abdul Rashid Aziz [2] and Michael Chia [1,*]

1. Physical Education and Sport Science Academic Group, National Institute of Education, Nanyang Technological University, Singapore 637616, Singapore; terence.chua@nie.edu.sg
2. Sport Medicine and Sport Science, Singapore Sport Institute, Singapore 397630, Singapore; abdul_rashid_aziz@sport.gov.sg
* Correspondence: michael.chia@nie.edu.sg

Received: 13 November 2020; Accepted: 10 December 2020; Published: 14 December 2020

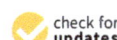

Abstract: We investigated whether a 4-min sprint interval training (SIT) protocol had an acute effect (15 min after) on improving alertness, mood, and memory recall in female students. Sixty-three children and 131 adolescents were randomly assigned to either a SIT or control (CON) group by the class Physical Education (PE) teachers. The SIT intervention was delivered twice a week for 3 weeks. SIT participants performed three, 20-s 'all-out' effort sprints interspersed with 60-s intervals of walking while CON group sat down and rested. PE lessons were arranged such that the first two sessions were to familiarise participants with the SIT protocol leading to acute assessments conducted on the third session. On that occasion, both groups rated their alertness and mood on a single-item hedonic scale and underwent an adapted memory recall test. The same assessments were administered to both groups fifteen minutes after delivery of SIT intervention. A 4-min SIT involving three, 20 s 'all-out' effort intensity sprints did not have an acute main effect on improving alertness, mood and, memory recall in female children ($\eta_p^2 = 0.009$) and adolescents ($\eta_p^2 = 0.012$). Students' exercise adherence and feedback from PE teachers are indicatives of the potential scalability of incorporating SIT into PE programmes. Different work-to-rest ratios could be used in future studies.

Keywords: sprint-interval training; learning in youths; acute exercise; school; attention

1. Introduction

Emergent literature suggests that a single session of aerobic exercise has beneficial effects on mood [1] and cognition [2] in adults. Reviews and meta-analyses have found that acute and chronic exercise improves attention and memory in children and adolescents [3,4]. These two domains of cognitive functions are essential for learning [5].

Improved cognition and enhanced mood after an acute bout of aerobic exercise may be explained by psychological and neurophysiological mechanisms. Exercise acts as an arousal stimulus [6]. Synthesis of brain-derived neurotropic factors (BDNF) is up-regulated leading to the activation of a pathway that initiates neuroplasticity and neurogenesis of the hippocampus [7,8]. Increased blood circulation during exercise also promotes more oxygen being delivered to the brain [9]. However, these underlying mechanisms are said to be dependent on exercise intensity. A meta-analysis revealed that studies utilising higher intensity exercise reported greater acute cognitive benefits [2]. The intensity of exercise can also affect mood differently [10]. Therefore, higher intensity exercise may be necessary for any potential positive effect on mood and cognition to be maximised. The acute and chronic exercise effects cannot be considered in isolation. It is explained that exercise training both in the short term (immediate and/or soon after) and long term (days, weeks, months, and years) increases the capacity for exercise, thereby permitting more vigorous and/or more prolonged individual exercise sessions and a more significant acute effect [11]. As such, an acute response to an exercise intervention refers to the transient effects of the exercise immediately or soon after the intervention.

Mood, alertness, and memory have facilitative influences on learning. These states of learning are different and but at the same time can be interdependent on each other. Young people experience a range of emotions, from positive emotions like enjoyment to negative emotions like anger, boredom, and anxiety in the process of learning. When negative emotions arise, learning may become a less enjoyable process to them. Consequently, they may be less motivated to interact with teachers and classmates [12,13]. The process of learning involves a continuous effort and awareness to inhibit the shift of attention to irrelevant activities [14,15]. Otherwise, a phenomenon called attentional bottleneck may manifest [16]. Children and adolescents spend six or more hours of their waking time in school, with much of those time spent engaging in sedentary activities due to classroom curriculum requirements and the inactive nature of most post-curriculum school-based activities [17]. Even though a single session of exercise is unlikely to cause impact on mood and cognition lasting throughout the schooling day, it may be opportunistic for qualified physical education teachers to enrich their students' formal learning experience by harvesting the immediate benefits of exercise.

The impact of interval training on cognition and learning in young people has generated research interest in recent years. Interval training can be characterized as sprint-interval training (SIT) or high-intensity interval training (HIIT). SIT involves very short bouts of 'all-out' effort sprints while HIIT involves relatively intense but submaximal workloads corresponding to 80–100% of maximal heart rate. Both forms of interval training are interspersed with periods of lower-intensity recovery [18]. Interval training resembles the sporadic patterns of physical play of free-living young people [19,20] and is generally well-tolerated [21,22]. The attractiveness of interval training is that the time invested to complete the exercise is only a fraction of that in traditional endurance training. This time-saving exercise modality is shown to be effective in improving cardiorespiratory fitness and certain cardiovascular and metabolic disease biomarkers in healthy and overweight youths when implemented as an exercise programme over several weeks to a few months [23–25].

Among various interval-training protocols that were studied in the literature, as little as three, 20 s all-out effort cycling sprints performed thrice a week for six weeks has shown to elicit chronic skeletal muscle adaptations linked to increased cardiorespiratory fitness as well as improved cardio-metabolic health biomarkers in adults [26]. This protocol involves a total work duration of 1 min. It is one of the shortest SIT methods to date to demonstrate positive health-related outcomes, albeit in adults. In terms of the acute effect of interval training on cognition in children and adolescents. Previous studies examining the acute effect of interval training on cognition in children and adolescents had used total work durations which were longer than that of Gillen and his colleagues' protocol. Some researchers used shorter intervals of exercise (10–20 s) while others used longer intervals of exercise (30 s) repeated between 8 and 16 times [27–29]. A 15- to 20-s bout of 'all-out' intensity sprint is suggested to be more palatable for children and adolescents rather than sprint bouts of longer durations (e.g., 30 s or 40 s) [30].

Interestingly, a recent study showed that embedding interval-training within the school day has led to increased moderate-intensity physical activity levels in adolescents [31]. Girls are oftentimes less active than boys [32–34] and hence the use of interval-training to increase physical activity has potential implications on them. Besides, girls are an under-served group compared to boys as research evidence in this area is scarce. Therefore, the primary objective of the study was to investigate the acute effect of a three, 20 s 'all-out' effort sprints on self-reported mood and alertness, and memory recall of female children and adolescents when delivered within a physical education (PE) setting. A secondary aim of the study was to gain perspectives from PE teachers about the feasibility of infusing SIT into physical education classes.

2. Materials and Methods

2.1. Enrolment of Participants and Institutional Ethical Clearance

One independent all-girl primary school and secondary school were invited to take part in the study via convenience sampling. The heads of PE department of both schools were contacts of the principal investigator. The school principal gave her consent and permission for conducting the research in schools was granted by the Ministry of Education. The study protocol and ethics was approved by the Institutional Review Board of the university on 4 April 2018 (IRB-2018-02-009-4). Upon discussion with the PE departments, one Primary 5 and one Secondary 1 cohorts were selected for the study. Written child assent and informed consent from the parents were obtained. Sixty-six female children (9–10 years old) and 131 female adolescents (12–13 years old) from the selected cohorts were enrolled in the study.

2.2. Study Design

The research employed a parallel, randomized control study design with a 1:1 allocation ratio. Participants were randomly assigned to either a SIT or control (CON) group at the individual level by the class PE teachers. The SIT intervention commenced twice a week for 3 weeks (6 sessions) and all PE lessons were conducted in the mornings, between 8 and 10 am. Following at least two separate familiarization sessions, the acute effects of SIT was assessed. Of the thirteen classes involved in the study, a few missed 1–2 SIT sessions due to timetabling constraints as reported by the respective PE teachers (i.e., PE lesson was cancelled when it fell on a public holiday).

2.3. SIT Protocol and Familiarisation Sessions Leading to the Day of Acute Assessment

The SIT group performed a three-minute warm-up routine (light lower limb stretches) followed by three 20 s 'all-out' effort running shuttle-sprints interspersed with intervals of 60 s of walking. The 3 × 20 s sprint bouts adapted from Gillen and his colleagues' work is one of the shortest SIT protocols to date. A work-to-rest ratio of 1:3 may be appropriate as a study showed that female children and adolescents were able to replicate the peak power generated in the first bout into subsequent bouts of the Wingate Anaerobic Test better than adult women [21]. This suggests that an active rest interval of 60 s derived from the 1:3 ratio may be sufficient for female children and adolescents to re-generate peak anaerobic power. The CON group did not receive the SIT intervention. Instead, they sat down and cheered on the SIT group during the shuttle sprints. Duration of the SIT protocol was four minutes and when warm-up was included, the total exercise session was less than eight minutes.

Prior to the study, the qualified PE teachers involved in the research were trained on how to deliver the SIT intervention and acute assessments by the principal investigator and his research assistant. The first two sessions were delivered to familiarise participants what an 'all-out' effort entails in the lead up to the acute assessments conducted on the third session. Each SIT participant was paired with a participant from the CON group who was tasked to count the number of sprint-shuttles completed over a marked out 20-m distance by their partner (data not presented). Upon the teacher's cue, the SIT group sprinted as hard as they could back and forth the marked-out distance for 20 s. Immediately after the 20 s sprint, participants walked to and from the marked-out distance for 60 s. With 15 s to go, participants were instructed to return to the starting position and get ready for the second bout. The process of a 20-s sprint bout followed by a 60-s walking recovery was repeated. Participants then performed their third and final bout of 20 s sprint and recovered right after for 60 s. Throughout the shuttle-sprints, partners of participants from the SIT group counted aloud the number of sprint shuttles completed and cheered the participants on to match or better the number of sprint shuttles completed in the previous bout. Most participants were able to match the number of shuttles completed in the previous sprint (data not reported). Indirectly, this indicated that participants were able to provide a maximal effort throughout the three sprint bouts.

2.4. Acute Assessment of Alertness, Mood, and Memory Recall (before and 15 min after SIT)

The primary outcome measures (i.e., alertness, mood, and memory recall) were assessed during the 3rd PE lesson. Before the SIT intervention was delivered, participants were asked to rate their mood and alertness from 1–10 on a mood scale [35] and a self-constructed alertness scale (i.e., higher number indicated better mood and greater alertness). The questions posed to them were: 'How are your mood right now? Please circle a number that best represents your current mood.' and 'How alert, watchful or attentive are you right now? Please circle a number that best describes you.' The scale consists of faces with expressions from frown to smiles above the number 1, 5, and 10 in gradations that are intended to reflect a progressive change of feelings. Hedonic scales like these are commonly administered to young children in consumer and food preference research. Although its psychometric properties for assessing mood and alertness are not established, another study has adapted it for the same purpose as the present study [31].

In addition, participants underwent an adapted version of the Rey Auditory Verbal Memory Recall test (RAVRT) [36]. The RAVRT was previously administered to the same age group of participants [37]. Instead of the full five trials, a single trial of recall was used in the present study. The PE teacher read out a list of 15 unrelated nouns each containing two syllables to the participants at a speed of one word per second. After the last word was read out, participants wrote down as many words as they could recall (order and spelling of words were not important). The number of correct words recalled by each participant was recorded. The RAVRT is commonly used in clinical research and practice and has a robust construct validity and internal consistency (Cronbach's alpha coefficient of 0.8) which was found to be closely associated with other tests of verbal learning which renders it to be a valid and reliable psychometric instrument.

Fifteen minutes after the SIT intervention was delivered, the same acute assessments were administered but in a different order. A different word list was used in the memory recall test of which the words are what students have learnt before. The delay of 11–20 min after exercise was reported to be the window of opportunity for observing the greatest positive effects on cognition. Positive effects may diminish beyond 20 min whereas assessing too soon after exercise may result in negative effects [2]. The study flow from enrolment of schools to data analysis of acute measures is shown in Figure 1 below.

At the end of the study, PE teachers were polled on their perceptions on the feasibility of incorporating SIT-type activities into their PE curriculum (i) to get students fit for sports and (ii) to get students healthy. The PE teachers provided their ratings on a self-constructed 5-point scale, with 1 being 'I do not find it feasible' and 5 being 'I find it very feasible'. To measure overall exercise adherence rate, the average percentage of the number of SIT participants who completed all SIT sessions was divided by the number of SIT participants in each class.

2.5. Statistical Analyses

SPSS Version 23 (IBM Corp., Armonk, NY, USA) was the statistical tool used. Normality of data and homogeneity of variance within each group was assessed. Missing data was replaced by series mean of each group. A 2 × 2 repeated-measures analysis of variance (ANOVA) was performed to analyse the main intervention effect. Given there were only two levels of measurements of the outcome variables (i.e., before condition and 15 min after condition), the assumption of sphericity was not violated. The measure of effect size was reported as partial eta square, where $\eta_p^2 = 0.01$–0.05 was interpreted as a small effect size, $\eta_p^2 = 0.06$–0.13 was interpreted as a medium effect size and $\eta_p^2 = 0.14$ or greater was interpreted as a large effect size. The level of statistical significance was determined as $p < 0.05$. Descriptive statistics (mean ± SD) for all outcome variables were reported.

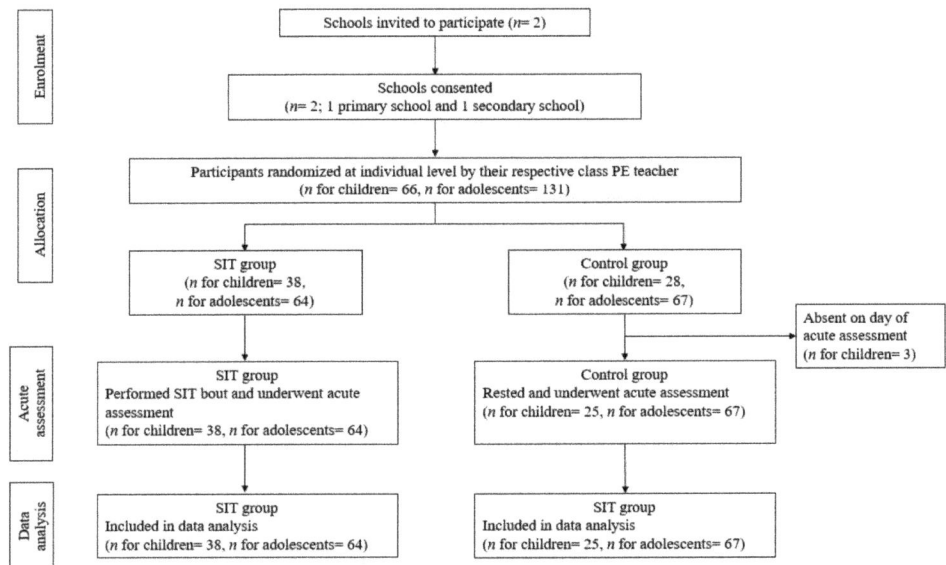

Figure 1. Flow diagram through each stage of the parallel, randomized control study design.

3. Results

3.1. Acute Changes in Self-Reported Alertness and Mood, and Memory Recall Score

Separate 2 × 2 repeated-measures ANOVAs were performed to compare the acute effect of a 4-min SIT protocol on improving alertness, mood, and memory recall with the CON group. The results of the univariate analysis of each outcome variable is presented in Table 1 for female children and in Table 2 for female adolescents. Multiple Analysis of Variance (MANOVA) revealed that there was no significant main effect of the SIT protocol on improving all three conditions of learning in female children, $F(3, 59) = 0.168$, $p = 0.918$, $\eta_p^2 = 0.008$, as well as in female adolescents, $F(3, 127) = 0.528$, $p = 0.664$, $\eta_p^2 = 0.012$. The time delay of 15 min following SIT has a significant effect on memory recall, with female children performing better ($F(1, 127) = 5.929$, $p = 0.018$, $\eta_p^2 = 0.089$) while female adolescents performed poorer ($F(1, 59) = 12.801$, $p = 0.001$, $\eta_p^2 = 0.09$) in the RAVRT after SIT. The pre-to-post-test change in self-reported alertness and mood, and memory recall scores between SIT and CON groups were not significantly different ($p > 0.05$). These results indicated that a four-minute SIT bout involving a combined one minute of 'all-out' effort sprints had no effect on improving alertness, mood, and memory recall in female children and adolescents.

3.2. Exercise Adherence and Teachers' Perceptions on Embedding SIT-Type Activities into the PE Curriculum

Most of the female participants (primary school children: 91.8 ± 5.0%, secondary school adolescents: 93.7 ± 9.2%) completed all SIT sessions that were delivered. Common reasons for their absenteeism reported by the class PE teachers were taking sick leave (not related to the exercise) and being out of school for inter-school competitions on the day of PE lesson. Six PE teachers involved in the study rated 4.2 and 4.0 (out of 5) on their beliefs in the feasibility of infusing SIT-type activities in their PE curriculum to get (i) students fit for sport and (ii) to keep students healthy, respectively. None of the participants were reported to have sustained injuries resulting from the 'all-out' intensity sprints under the tutelage of the qualified PE teachers.

Table 1. Mean ± SD of alertness, mood, and memory recall of female primary school children.

	SIT Group (n = 38)			Control Group (n = 25)			Effect size of changes between groups, η_p^2	Repeated Measures ANOVA		
	Pre-exercise	11–20 min post-exercise	Change	Pre-intervention	11–20 min post-condition	Change		Time (p-value)	Group (p-value)	Time* group (p-value)
Alertness	6.9 ± 2.1	6.8 ± 2.5	−0.1	6.9 ± 1.7	6.6 ± 1.1	−0.3	0.001	0.353	0.884	0.632
Mood	6.2 ± 2.4	6.1 ± 2.0	−0.1	6.2 ± 2.1	6.6 ± 1.7	0.4	0.006	0.671	0.545	0.360
Memory recall	6.5 ± 1.8	7.6 ± 2.1	1.1	7.0 ± 2.0	7.3 ± 1.7	0.3	0.001	0.018	0.927	0.177

* Interaction between time of assessment and experimental group.

Table 2. Mean ± SD of alertness, mood, and memory recall of female secondary school adolescents.

	SIT Group (n = 64)			Control Group (n = 67)			Effect size of changes between groups, η_p^2	Repeated Measures ANOVA		
	Pre-exercise	11–20 min post-exercise	Change	Pre-intervention	11–20 min post-condition	Change		Time (p-value)	Group (p-value)	Time* group (p-value)
Alertness	6.1 ± 1.5	6.1 ± 1.5	0	6.0 ± 2.1	5.9 ± 1.9	−0.1	0.003	0.687	0.556	0.534
Mood	6.1 ± 1.5	6.0 ± 1.6	−0.1	5.7 ± 2.2	5.7 ± 2.0	0	0.11	0.745	0.237	0.442
Memory recall	10.5 ± 2.2	9.9 ± 2.2	−0.6	10.8 ± 2.2	10.0 ± 2.3	−0.8	0.001	0.001	0.825	0.707

* Interaction between time of assessment and experimental group.

4. Discussion

The primary objective of the study was to examine the acute effect of a SIT protocol involving three, 20-s 'all-out' effort sprints on improving mood, alertness and memory recall in female primary school children and secondary school adolescents. Of interest was also the PE teachers' perspectives on using SIT in a lesson setting (i.e., teachers' thoughts on infusing SIT-type activity in PE lessons as an intervention to get students fit for sports and keeping students healthy). The key findings of the present study were that a 4-min SIT protocol involving three-, 20 s 'all-out' effort sprint did not have any acute effect on self-reported mood, alertness, and memory recall in female children and adolescents. These results did not support the authors' hypothesis that very brief interval exercise enhances student states of learning. Contrary to the present results, previous studies showed that school-based interval training elicited a positive impact on student alertness. A programme called FUNtervals, a six-minute interval exercise that involved four minutes of dynamic, whole-body exercises such as squats, jumping jacks and running on the spot performed at high-intensity showed acute improvements in selective attention in 88 boys and girls aged 9–11 years [29]. In the cited study, the children made fewer errors in the d2 test, an objective measure of one's selective attention, following the FUNtervals session compared to when they were being assigned to a no-activity break group. This was apparently the only study that examined the effects of HIIT following a brief delay of 11–20 min, as in the present study. It was previously suggested in a meta-analysis that a post-exercise delay of 11–20 min was most likely to elicit positive responses in cognition [2]. Interestingly, a recent study reported that the boost in selective attention in 158 adolescents lasted for an hour after a 16-min HIIT session [38]. The 12- to 16-year-old adolescents in the cited study were instructed to perform 30 s of high-intensity exercise in between rest intervals of 30 s.

Findings in the literature on the effect of school-based interval training on mood in children and adolescents are scarce. The SIT protocol in the present study used only one movement task, that is sprinting, rather than a series of different body movements. By the day of acute assessment, the activity became rather mundane to the participants as commented by one of the PE teachers. This could have dampened their motivation and resulted in the lack of change in their self-reported affect. This view concurred with previous findings from Cooper and his colleagues who reported that 10 × 10 s running sprints, interspersed with 50 s of active recovery had no beneficial immediate effect on self-reported energy, tension, and calmness in adolescents [27]. Participants in the cited study reported a higher level of tiredness following the exercise than when they were seated in the resting trial. It is likely that participants' mood was in an attenuated state when the mood questionnaire was administered soon after exercise. These results were in contrast with findings reported by another study [28]. They reported that the mood of 21 adolescents improved significantly following an eight- to 10-min HIIT intervention. The reasons for such mixed results are not readily apparent but differences in interval-training protocols, participant cohorts, and the timings of the assessments are plausible explanations.

Few studies have investigated the acute effect of HIIT on memory recall in children or adolescents. Findings in the present study showed negligible effect on memory recall in both primary school children and secondary school adolescents. Similarly, no acute effect on visuo-spatial memory and pictorial memory recall in adolescents were reported in other studies [27,38]. Instead, researchers in the latter cited study showed that selective attention and concentration increased in the second and third hour after the HIIT intervention. It is noteworthy that the HIIT protocol employed in the cited study is four times the duration (16 versus 4 min) of the SIT protocol used in the present study. The interval training protocols used in the cited studies were not identical to that used in the present study. (i.e., work-to-rest ratio; total exercise time). In addition, differing qualitative characteristics of the movement tasks (i.e., cognitive demand and coordinative complexity) may have accounted for the mixed results. It was suggested that activity that requires greater attentional and cognitive resources led to greater extent of improvement in cognition than activities with low cognitive engagement [39,40]. The movement task used in the present study is sprinting which most children and adolescents are quite accustomed to. It also does not require a greater degree of coordination compared to exercises described in other studies. Combining the results of 6 acute studies, the authors of a recent review had found that a single bout of HIIT produced significant yet small to moderate acute effects on executive function and affect in youths [41]. Therefore, whether such brief interval training interventions are useful need to be addressed using different perspectives in different school contexts. For instance, the efficacy of SIT-type programmes that are time-saving and low volume in helping female youths adopt a less sedentary lifestyle outside of school.

The use of a single-item hedonic scale is reported elsewhere and is also used for self-reporting purposes in adolescents [28]. Adolescents in the cited study were asked to complete the hedonic mood scale before and after every HIIT session throughout the period of intervention (a total of 24 times). In contrast to the present findings, adolescents' mood following HIIT significantly improved by an average of 0.97. Unlike other questionnaires used in the interval training literature, the single-item hedonic mood scale is not established as a validated instrument. Notwithstanding its unestablished validity, the single-item hedonic scale takes less than one minute to answer and is easily comprehensible to children and adolescents.

The total time taken to complete the SIT protocol in the present study is a fraction of the time taken by participants in other studies cited in the literature—i.e., 4 min in present study vs. 10 and 16 min in other studies [27,38]. It is plausible that the exercise dose in the present study was too brief to have any effect on alertness, mood, and memory recall from baseline values (pre-SIT intervention). In the present study, participants reported they were relatively alert and in good mood, and their memory recall scores were not markedly in deficit before the acute SIT intervention. The absence of significant difference is plausibly due to a ceiling effect for improvement [42] since PE sessions were conducted relatively early in the morning of a schooling day where children and adolescents are reasonably rested.

4.1. Exercise Adherence and PE Teachers' Perspective on Infusing SIT in PE Classes

The qualified PE teachers who conducted the study were specially trained by the principal investigator and his team. To motivate participants to perform 'all-out' intensity efforts, they were encouraged to match or better the number of sprint-shuttles completed in the previous bouts. Although the proportion of participants who managed to match or better their number of sprint-shuttles is not reported in the present study, a majority had completed all SIT sessions conducted (91.8% and 93.7% of the female children and adolescents, respectively). The exercise adherence in the present study compares well with the exercise adherence rate of 90% among Australian adolescents reported elsewhere [43]. The continued participation even after the third session, when acute assessment of alertness, mood and memory recall were administered, is an indication that SIT is an appealing exercise for female children and adolescents in the context of the present study. Additionally, when PE teachers were asked for their perceptions on the feasibility in incorporating SIT-type activities in PE lessons, ratings provided were very encouraging. Like the present study, several studies had situated the delivery of interval training as an exercise intervention during PE classes, albeit for different purposes [44]. On the balance of discussion, it appears that PE classes could be avenues where SIT-type or HIIT-type activities can feature, given its flexibility in incorporating different forms of dynamic exercise movements as well as its time-saving regimen.

4.2. Strengths and Limitations of Study

A unique contribution of the present study was that it involved a cohort entirely of female participants and was one of the largest cross-sectional study that the authors are aware of. Furthermore, the high retention rate and positive ratings from PE teachers are indications of the potential scalability of introducing SIT-type programme in schools. A limitation of the present study was that the acute assessments for mood, alertness, and memory recall were measured on only one occasion and specifically within the period of 11–20 min (i.e., about 15 min) after the SIT. It is indeterminate in the present study if the prescribed SIT protocol has any abbreviated or transient effect on the aforementioned factors that affects learning outside of the 11- to 20-min window. In addition, as this study was conducted only on female participants, the effect of SIT on male participants remains to be examined.

4.3. Future Research Directions

Future research could explore different permutations on the work-to-rest ratio of the SIT protocol and examine its acute effect on mood, alertness, and memory recall of children and adolescents in a school-based setting. Interval-training could be embedded during the latter part of a school day when mood, alertness and memory of students are on the wane. These brief exercise breaks should be low in volume so that it does not take up much of class time and they should be curated with participant enjoyment in mind.

5. Conclusions

A 4-min SIT involving three, 20 s 'all-out' effort intensity sprints had no acute effect on improving mood, alertness and memory in female children and adolescents. The high exercise adherence rate and encouraging ratings by PE teachers are suggestive of the potential scalability of incorporating SIT into PE programme in schools. There is a need for more school-based research to explore the acute effect of different SIT permutations in the context of each school.

Author Contributions: T.C.: Research coordination, data collection & analysis, manuscript writing; A.R.A.: Study co-conception, manuscript review and revision; M.C.: Research oversight, study conception, manuscript writing, grant owner. All authors have read and agreed to the published version of the manuscript.

Funding: This research was supported by the National Institute of Education, Singapore, under the RS-SAA institutional grant (reference no. RS 6/17 MC).

Acknowledgments: The authors would like to acknowledge the school principals, teachers in the physical education departments and participants of both schools for their support, involvement and participation in the study.

Conflicts of Interest: The authors declare no potential conflict of interest.

Availability of data and material: Data used in the manuscript will be deposited to the data repository of the corresponding author's institution. Permission from the corresponding author before accessing the data is required.

References

1. Guszkowska, M. Effects of exercise on anxiety, depression and mood. *Psychiatr. Pol.* **2004**, *38*, 611–620. [PubMed]
2. Chang, Y.K.; Labban, J.D.; Gapin, J.I.; Etnier, J.L. The effects of acute exercise on cognitive performance: A meta-analysis. *Brain Res.* **2012**, *1453*, 87–101. [CrossRef] [PubMed]
3. de Greeff, J.W.; Bosker, R.J.; Oosterlaan, J.; Visscher, C.; Hartman, E. Effects of physical activity on executive functions, attention and academic performance in preadolescent children: A meta-analysis. *J. Sci. Med. Sport* **2018**, *21*, 501–507. [CrossRef] [PubMed]
4. Li, J.W.; O'Connor, H.; O'Dwyer, N.; Orr, R. The effect of acute and chronic exercise on cognitive function and academic performance in adolescents: A systematic review. *J. Sci. Med. Sport* **2017**, *20*, 841–848. [CrossRef] [PubMed]
5. Ylikrekola, A.; Särelä, J.; Valpola, H. Selective attention improves learning. In *Artificial Neural Networks–ICANN 2009, Proceedings of the 19th International Conference, Limassol, Cyprus, 14–17 September 2009*; Springer: Munich, Germany; pp. 285–294.
6. Christiansen, L.; Beck, M.M.; Bilenberg, N.; Wienecke, J.; Astrup, A.; Lundbye-Jensen, J. Effects of exercise on cognitive performance in children and adolescents with ADHD: Potential mechanisms and evidence-based recommendations. *J. Clin. Med.* **2019**, *8*, 841. [CrossRef]
7. Vaynman, S.; Ying, Z.; Gomez-Pinilla, F. Hippocampal BDNF mediates the efficacy of exercise on synaptic plasticity and cognition. *Eur. J. Neurosci.* **2004**, *20*, 2580–2590. [CrossRef]

8. Wrann, C.D.; White, J.P.; Salogiannnis, J.; Laznik-Bogoslavski, D.; Wu, J.; Ma, D.; Lin, J.D.; Greenberg, M.E.; Spiegelman, B.M. Exercise induces hippocampal BDNF through a PGC-1α/FNDC5 pathway. *Cell Metab.* **2013**, *18*, 649–659. [CrossRef]
9. Querido, J.S.; Sheel, A.W. Regulation of Cerebral Blood Flow During Exercise. *Sports Med.* **2007**, *37*, 765–782. [CrossRef]
10. Kennedy, M.M.; Newton, M. Effect of exercise intensity on mood in step aerobics. *J. Sports Med. Phys. Fit.* **1997**, *37*, 200–204.
11. Thompson, P.D.; Crouse, S.F.; Goodpaster, B.; Kelley, D.; Moyna, N.; Pescatello, L. The acute versus the chronic response to exercise. *Med. Sci. Sports Exerc.* **2001**, *33*, S438–S453. [CrossRef]
12. Pekrun, R.; Goetz, T.; Titz, W.; Perry, R.P. Academic emotions in students' self-regulated learning and achievement: A program of qualitative and quantitative research. *Educ. Psychol.* **2002**, *37*, 91–105. [CrossRef]
13. Trezise, K.; University of Melbourne, Melbourne, Victoria, Australia; Bourgeois, A. (The University of Queensland, Brisbane, Queensland, Australia); Luck, C. (Curtin University, Perth, Western Australia, Australia). Personal communication, 2017. Emotions in classrooms: The need to understand how emotions Affect and education.
14. Hobbis, M. (University College London, London, United Kingdom, England). Personal communication, 2017. We should pay attention to attention.
15. Ko, L.W.; Komarov, O.; Hairston, W.D.; Jung, T.-P.; Lin, C.-T. Sustained Attention in Real Classroom Settings: An EEG Study. *Front. Hum. Neurosci.* **2017**, *11*. [CrossRef]
16. Atkinson, R.C.; Shiffrin, R.M. Human memory: A proposed system and its control processes. In *The Psychology of Learning and Motivation*; Spence, K.W., Spence, J.T., Eds.; Academic Press: New York, NY, USA, 1968; Volume 2, pp. 89–195.
17. Lye, J.C.T.; Mukherjee, S.; Chia, M.H.Y. Physical activity and sedentary behavior patterns of Singaporean adolescents. *J. Phys. Act. Health* **2015**, *12*, 1213–1220.
18. Weston, K.S.; Wisløff, U.; Coombes, J.S. High-intensity interval training in patients with lifestyle-induced cardiometabolic disease: A systematic review and meta-analysis. *Br. J. Sports Med.* **2014**, *48*, 1227–1234. [CrossRef] [PubMed]
19. Bailey, R.C.; Olson, J.O.D.I.; Pepper, S.L.; Porszasz, J.A.N.O.S.; Barstow, T.J.; Cooper, D.M. The level and tempo of children's physical activities: An observational study. *Med. Sci. Sports Exerc.* **1995**, *27*, 1033–1041. [CrossRef] [PubMed]
20. Howe, C.A.; Freedson, P.S.; Feldman, H.A.; Osganian, S.K. Energy expenditure and enjoyment of common children's games in a simulated free-play environment. *J. Pediatr.* **2010**, *15*, 936–942. [CrossRef]
21. Chia, M. Power recovery in the Wingate Anaerobic Test in girls and women following prior sprints of a short duration. *Biol. Sport* **2001**, *18*, 45–53.
22. De Araujo, A.C.C.; Roschel, H.; Picanço, A.R.; do Prado, D.M.L.; Villares, S.M.F.; de Sa Pinto, A.L.; Gualano, B. Similar health benefits of endurance and high-intensity interval training in obese children. *PLoS ONE* **2012**, *7*, e42747. [CrossRef]
23. Cockcroft, E.J.; Bond, B.; Williams, C.A.; Harris, S.; Jackman, S.R.; Armstrong, N.; Barker, A.R. The effects of two weeks high-intensity interval training on fasting glucose, glucose tolerance and insulin resistance in adolescent boys: A pilot study. *BMC Sports Sci. Med. Rehabil.* **2019**, *11*, 29. [CrossRef]
24. Eddolls, W.T.; McNarry, M.A.; Stratton, G.; Winn, C.O.; Mackintosh, K.A. High-intensity interval training interventions in children and adolescents: A systematic review. *Sports Med.* **2017**, *47*, 2363–2374. [CrossRef]
25. Thivel, D.; Masurier, J.; Baquet, G.; Timmons, B.W.; Pereira, B.; Berthoin, S.; Duclos, M.; Aucouturier, J. High-intensity interval training in overweight and obese children and adolescents: Systematic review and meta-analysis. *J. Sports Med. Phys. Fit.* **2019**, *59*, 310–324. [CrossRef] [PubMed]
26. Gillen, J.B.; Percival, M.E.; Skelly, L.E.; Martin, B.J.; Tan, R.B.; Tarnopolsky, M.A.; Gibala, M. Three minutes of all-out intermittent exercise per week increases skeletal muscle oxidative capacity and improves cardiometabolic health. *PLoS ONE* **2014**, *9*, e111489. [CrossRef] [PubMed]
27. Cooper, S.B.; Bandelow, S.; Nute, M.L.; Dring, K.J.; Stannard, R.L.; Morris, J.G.; Nevill, M.E. Sprint-based exercise and cognitive function in adolescents. *Prev. Med. Rep.* **2016**, *4*, 155–161. [CrossRef] [PubMed]
28. Costigan, S.A.; Eather, N.; Plotnikoff, R.C.; Hillman, C.H.; Lubans, D.R. High-intensity interval training on cognitive and mental health in adolescents. *Med. Sci. Sports Exerc.* **2016**, *48*, 1985–1993. [CrossRef]

29. Ma, J.K.; Le Mare, L.; Gurd, B.J. Four minutes of in-class high-intensity interval activity improves selective attention in 9-to 11-year olds. *Appl. Physiol. Nutr. Metab.* **2014**, *40*, 238–244. [CrossRef]
30. Chia, M.; Armstrong, N.; Childs, D. The assessment of children's anaerobic performance using modifications of the Wingate anaerobic test. *Pediatr. Exerc. Sci.* **1997**, *9*, 80–89. [CrossRef]
31. Costigan, S.A.; Ridgers, N.D.; Eather, N.; Plotnikoff, R.C.; Harris, N.; Lubans, D.R. Exploring the impact of high intensity interval training on adolescents' objectively measured physical activity: Findings from a randomized controlled trial. *J. Sports Sci.* **2018**, *36*, 1087–1094. [CrossRef]
32. Chia, M. Pedometer-assessed physical activity of Singaporean youths. *Prev. Med.* **2010**, *50*, 262–264. [CrossRef]
33. Duncan, J.S.; Schofield, G.; Duncan, E.K. Pedometer-determined physical activity and body composition in New Zealand children. *Med. Sci. Sports Exerc.* **2006**, *38*, 1402–1409. [CrossRef]
34. Duncan, M.J.; Al-Nakeeb, Y.; Woodfield, L.; Lyons, M. Pedometer determined physical activity levels in primary school children from Central England. *Prev. Med.* **2007**, *44*, 416–420. [CrossRef]
35. Ottawa Mood Scale. Available online: http://www.drcheng.ca/resources/Articles/mood_scales-facesforallages.pdf (accessed on 13 November 2020).
36. Rey, A. *Clinical Tests in Psychology [In French]*; Presses Universitaires de France: Paris, France, 1964.
37. Wong, P.; Boh, G.B.T.; Wang, J.C.K.; Chia, M.Y.H. Relationship between obesity and verbal memory performance among top academic achievers in Singapore. *Asian J. Exerc. Sports Sci.* **2007**, *4*, 47–55.
38. Mezcua-Hidalgo, A.; Ruiz-Ariza, A.; Suárez-Manzano, S.; Martínez-López, E.J. 48-Hour Effects of Monitored Cooperative High-Intensity Interval Training on Adolescent Cognitive Functioning. *Percept. Mot. Ski.* **2019**, *126*, 202–222. [CrossRef] [PubMed]
39. Pesce, C. Shifting the focus from quantitative to qualitative exercise characteristics in exercise and cognition research. *J. Sport Exerc. Psychol.* **2012**, *34*, 766–786. [CrossRef] [PubMed]
40. Vazou, S.; Pesce, C.; Lakes, K.; Smiley-Oyen, A. More than one road leads to Rome: A narrative review and meta-analysis of physical activity intervention effects on cognition in youth. *Int. J. Sport Exerc. Psychol.* **2019**, *17*, 153–178. [CrossRef] [PubMed]
41. Leahy, A.A.; Mavilidi, M.F.; Smith, J.J.; Hillman, C.H.; Eather, N.; Barker, D.; Lubans, D.R. Review of High-Intensity Interval Training for Cognitive and Mental Health in Youth. *Med. Sci. Sports Exerc.* **2020**, *52*, 2224–2234. [CrossRef] [PubMed]
42. Hessling, R.M.; Traxel, N.M.; Schmidt, T.J. Ceiling effect. In *The SAGE Encyclopedia of Social Science Research Methods*; Lewis-Beck, M.S., Bryman, A., Liao, T.F., Eds.; Sage Publications Inc.: Thousand Oaks, CA, USA, 2004. [CrossRef]
43. Leahy, A.; Hillman, C.; Shigeta, T.; Smith, J.; Eather, N.; Morgan, P.; Plotnikoff, R.; Nilsson, M.; Lonsdale, C.; Noetel, M. Teacher facilitated high-intensity interval training intervention for older adolescents: The 'Burn 2 Learn' pilot randomised controlled trial. *J. Sci. Med. Sport* **2018**, *21*, S72. [CrossRef]
44. Zapata-Lamana, R.; Cuevas, I.C.; Fuentes, V.; Soto Espindola, C.; Romero, P.E.; Sepulveda, C.; Monsalves-Alvarez, M. HIITing Health in School: Can High Intensity Interval Training Be a Useful and Reliable Tool for Health on a School-Based Environment? A Systematic Review. *Int. J. Sch. Health* **2019**, *6*, 1–10. [CrossRef]

Publisher's Note: MDPI stays neutral with regard to jurisdictional claims in published maps and institutional affiliations.

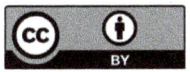

© 2020 by the authors. Licensee MDPI, Basel, Switzerland. This article is an open access article distributed under the terms and conditions of the Creative Commons Attribution (CC BY) license (http://creativecommons.org/licenses/by/4.0/).

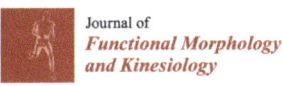

Article

The Prevalence of Urinary Incontinence among Adolescent Female Athletes: A Systematic Review

Tamara Rial Rebullido [1], Cinta Gómez-Tomás [2,*], Avery D. Faigenbaum [3] and Iván Chulvi-Medrano [4]

1. Tamara Rial Exercise & Women's Health, Newtown, PA 18790, USA; rialtamara@gmail.com
2. Research Group Physiotherapy and Readaptation in Sport, Department of Physiotherapy, Catholic University of Murcia (UCAM), 3010 Murcia, Spain
3. Department of Health and Exercise Science, The College of New Jersey, Ewing, NJ 08628, USA; faigenba@tcnj.edu
4. UIRFIDE (Sport Performance and Physical Fitness Research Group), Department of Physical and Sports Education, Faculty of Physical Activity and Sports Sciences, University of Valencia, 46010 Valencia, Spain; ivan.chulvi@uv.es
* Correspondence: mariacintagomez@gmail.com

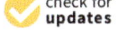

Citation: Rebullido, T.R.; Gómez-Tomás, C.; Faigenbaum, A.D.; Chulvi-Medrano, I. The Prevalence of Urinary Incontinence among Adolescent Female Athletes: A Systematic Review. *J. Funct. Morphol. Kinesiol.* **2021**, *6*, 12. https://doi.org/10.3390/jfmk6010012

Academic Editor: Cristina Cortis
Received: 5 January 2021
Accepted: 24 January 2021
Published: 28 January 2021

Publisher's Note: MDPI stays neutral with regard to jurisdictional claims in published maps and institutional affiliations.

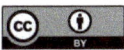

Copyright: © 2021 by the authors. Licensee MDPI, Basel, Switzerland. This article is an open access article distributed under the terms and conditions of the Creative Commons Attribution (CC BY) license (https://creativecommons.org/licenses/by/4.0/).

Abstract: This review aimed to synthesize the most up-to-date evidence regarding the prevalence of urinary incontinence (UI) among adolescent female athletes. We conducted a systematic review of studies regarding UI in female athletes less than 19 years of age. This review was conducted in accordance with the Preferred Reporting Items for Systematic Reviews and Meta-analyses (PRIMSA). The electronic databases of PubMed, Embase, Cochrane Central Register of Controlled Trials (CENTRAL), Scopus, and Web of Science (WOS) were searched between October and November 2020. After blinded peer evaluation, a total of 215 studies were identified and nine were included. Risk of bias was assessed using the Strengthening the Reporting of Observational Studies in Epidemiology (STROBE) checklist. This review identified a prevalence of UI in adolescent female athletes between 18% to 80% with an average of 48.58%. The most prevalent sports were trampolining followed by rope skipping. The prevalence of UI among adolescent female athletes practicing impact sports was significantly prevalent. There is a need for further research, education, and targeted interventions for adolescent female athletes with UI.

Keywords: pelvic floor dysfunction; women's health; pelvic floor training; youth

1. Introduction

Urinary incontinence (UI) is defined as any complaint of involuntary loss of urine [1]. Mostly prevalent in women, the broad range of UI is 5–27% [2], with an average prevalence of 27.6% based on a review of population studies [3]. The most common type of UI is stress urinary incontinence (SUI) that is defined as any complaint of involuntary loss of urine on effort or physical exertion [1]. Strenuous exercise has been cited as a risk factor for developing symptoms of SUI [4]. Recently, a subcategory of athletic incontinence was proposed as a new term for a specific SUI that occurs during sport activities or competition [5]. One of the most prevalent pelvic floor dysfunctions reported in female athletes is SUI [6–9]. For instance, a meta-analysis that included 7507 women with age ranges between 12 and 69 years, found that the prevalence of SUI was 33.69% for the female athletes compared to 24.40% in the control group [10].

The younger female athletes seem to display isolated symptoms of pure stress UI which is an uncomplicated SUI without other symptoms of urge incontinence or bladder dysfunction [11]. High-impact sports involving jumping, landing or running have shown the highest prevalence rates of urinary loss among young female athletes [12–15]. A recent meta-analysis by Teixeira et al. found a 35% prevalence rate of UI in female athletes (average age of 23.8 years) practicing different sports. When compared with sedentary women, female athletes displayed a 177% higher risk of presenting with UI symptoms [16]. Moreover, female athletes practicing high-intensity activities displayed greater odd ratios of SUI symptoms than those practicing less intense physical activity [9,17]. Similar UI prevalence rates (25.9%) were described in a review with meta-analysis focusing on female athletes involved in high-impact sports such as volleyball, athletics, basketball, cross-country, skiing, and running [8]. UI during practice or competition can cause embarrassment and negatively impact athletic performance. It has been reported that a vast majority of female athletes (~80%) with UI are too embarrassed to tell their coaches, which sustains unawareness of the problem and delays intervention [18,19]. UI can affect an athlete's quality of life and impact performance [20], leading to sport drop-out [15,21].

The underlying mechanisms by which young nulliparous female athletes show higher levels of UI as compared to their sedentary females [16,17] are still not scientifically understood. The continence mechanism during sports practice has been hypothesized to be affected by a variety of kinematic and sport-related factors such as pelvic floor displacement during jumps and running [22,23], neuromuscular fatigue of the pelvic floor muscles during strenuous physical activity [24], and morphological changes of the pelvic floor muscles [25]. Moreover, low energy availability, low body mass index (BMI), estrogen changes, and hypermobility joint syndrome have also been suggested as possible contributing factors for developing UI in female athletes [26,27].

Elite female athletes experiencing UI at an early stage are more likely to report UI symptoms later in life [7]. This is a condition that should be addressed early in life and studied in order to provide better care and support. To date, little is known about the pelvic floor function of young female athletes. Although previous systematic reviews have analyzed the incidence of UI in physically active and athletic females of all ages [4,8,10,16], no previous reports have focused their attention on adolescent female athletes. Given the unique developmental characteristics occurring during adolescence and the previously demonstrated association between high impact training and UI, the prevalence of UI in adolescent athletes needs to be specifically addressed. Our main goal was to identify the prevalence of UI in female athletes less than 19 years of age and provide an understanding of the types of sports associated with the highest prevalence rates.

2. Materials and Methods

2.1. Information Sources and Search

The conduct and reporting of this systematic review complied with the Preferred Reporting Items for Systematic review and Meta-Analyses (PRISMA) guidelines [28].

A systematic search of electronic databases including PubMed, Embase, Cochrane Central Register of Controlled Trials (CENTRAL), Scopus, and Web of Science (WOS) was carried out between October and November 2020 independently by two blinded authors. No restrictions on language or publication timeline were applied. The search strategy used keywords, mesh terms, and Boolean connectors (AND/OR) including: "Stress urinary incontinence" OR "urine loss" OR "pelvic floor muscles" AND sport OR athlete OR "female athlete". Search results were limited to species (human) and age (birth–18 years) and source type (journals).

2.2. Eligibility Criteria and Study Selection

Retrieved titles and abstracts were assessed for eligibility for inclusion, and duplicate entries were removed. The same two authors independently reviewed the text of the studies for eligibility. Articles published up to November 2020 were eligible for inclusion. The criteria for inclusion were: (1) study participants included adolescent females participating in sport or athletic activities; (2) study provides an assessment of UI symptoms; (3) study published in a peer-reviewed journal in any language. Randomized controlled trials (RCTs) with two or more parallel groups and crossover trials, non-RCTs were eligible for inclusion if they met the previously mentioned criteria. The criteria for study exclusion were: (1) participants > 19 years old; (2) participants who underwent any type of pelvic floor surgery; (3) participants during their pregnancy and postpartum period and; (4) systematic review, meta-analysis, or case study.

2.3. Data Collection Process and Quality Assessment

For each study, data were extracted on the characteristics of the population and intervention such as: (1) last name of the first author; (2) years of publication; (3) study design; (4) sample characteristics (age, sample analyzed, weight, body mass index, sport practice, and hours of weekly training); and (5) instrument assessing symptoms of UI. Risk of bias was assessed independently by two authors using the Strengthening the Reporting of Observational Studies in Epidemiology (STROBE) checklist [29]. The same two researchers rated the studies and discrepancies were resolved by consensus. Data reporting completeness was assessed by applying the STROBE cross-sectional checklist reporting classified as "not reported or unclear", "some information mentioned but insufficient", or "clear and detailed information provided".

3. Results

3.1. Study Selection

The search strategy yielded 500 potentially relevant studies. After the removal of duplicates, 321 records were screened. Of those, 215 potential titles were selected after the database filter insertion. Among those, only nine studies met the criteria for inclusion and were selected for analysis in this systematic review. The study selection flow chart is shown in Figure 1.

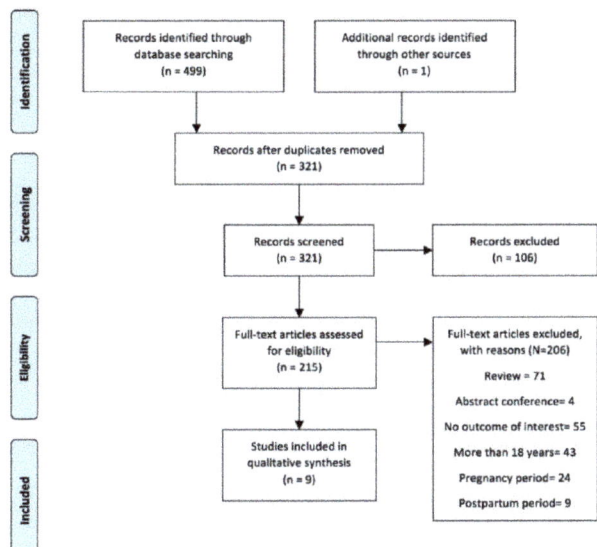

Figure 1. Flow diagram for the study selection.

3.2. Overview of Study Characteristics

Table 1 provides an overview of the characteristics of the studies included in this review. Table 2 provides the participants' characteristics of weight, body mass index (BMI), and hours of training per week.

Table 1. Summary of the studies included in this review.

Authors, Year	Study	Sample Size	Mean Age (Range or SD)	Sport	Grade Impact * Based on Criteria [30]	Main Outcome (UI Tools)	% UI	Secondary Outcomes	Secondary Outcomes Results
Eliasson et al., 2002 [31].	Cross-sectional	$n = 35$	15 (12–22)	Trampoline	3	Pad-weighting test	80 mean leakage of 28 g	Muscular strength with perineometer	23 of 27 diodes on the perineometer for 6 s and 20 for 30 s, 30 cm H_2O of intravaginal squeeze pressure
Carls et al., 2007 [18]	Cross-sectional	$n = 86$	17 (14–21)	High impact sports	3	The Bristol Female Lower Urinary Tract Symptoms Questionnaire	28	Educational prevention and treatment of UI	90% had never heard of pelvic muscle exercises (Kegels)
Parmigiano et al., 2014 [19]	Cross-sectional	$n = 148$	15 (2.0)	Soccer, handball, basketball, wrestling, judo, track and field, swimming, boxing	2,3	Pre-participation gynecological examination (PPGE)	Total = 18.2 Track and Field = 14.30; Basketball = 8.30; Boxing = 25; Soccer= 11.60; Handball = 6.40; Judo = 33.30; Swimming = 16.70	Eating attitudes test	15% risk of eating disorders; 89.9% were not familiar with the occurrence of UI in athletes; 87.1% would not mention to coach.
Fernandes et al., 2014 [32]	Cross-sectional	$n = 35$	15.6 (12–19)	Soccer	2	Urinary Incontinence short form (ICIQ-UI SF)	62.8	The pad test and King's Health Questionnaire (KHQ)	35.2 score in the General Health domain; 37.3 in the emotions domain; 26.5 in the Sleep/Energy domain.
Da Roza et al., 2015 [33]	Cross-sectional	$n = 22$	18.1 (3.4)	Trampoline	3	Urinary Incontinence short form (ICIQ-UI SF)	72.7	Amount of urinary loss, frequency of involuntary loss	93.7% self-classified as moderate amount of UI; frequency of UI once a week or less.
Almeida et al., 2015 [34]	Cross-sectional	$n = 67$	18 (5)	Volleyball, judo, gymnastics, trampoline, swimming	2,3	Urinary Incontinence short form (ICIQ-UI SF)	Total = 52.2 Volleyball = 43.5; Trampoline = 88.9; Swimming = 50; Judo = 44.4	Fecal Incontinence Severity Index, Female Sexual Function Index, vaginal symptoms and pelvic organ prolapse symptoms (ICIQ-VS)	Involuntary loss of gas: 64.6% athletes, 58.5% nonathletes; POP: 0% athletes, 2% nonathletes; dyspareunia: 13.8% athletes, 21.9% nonathletes; 31.4% athlete's strategy: "Emptying the bladder before training"; 52.0% nonathlete's strategy: "Emptying the bladder before leaving the house".

Table 1. *Cont.*

Authors, Year	Study	Sample Size	Mean Age (Range or SD)	Sport	Grade Impact * Based on Criteria [30]	Main Outcome (UI Tools)	% UI	Secondary Outcomes	Secondary Outcomes Results
Logan et al., 2017 [14]	Pilot study: Cross-sectional	n = 44	(13–17)	Cross-country, track and field, field-hockey, soccer	2,3	Urinary Incontinence short form (ICIQ-UI-SF)	48	Identify risk factor	32% vigorous exercise, 34% during laughter, 14% activities of daily living (ADLs).
Dobrowolski et al., 2019 [12]	Cross-sectional	n = 89	16 (15–21) *	Rope skipping	3	Prevalence of SUI 11-point Likert scale (0–10)	75	Quality of life (ICIQ-SF), non-validated sport-specific questionnaire inspired by (IIQ-7)	21% indicated an overall interference of SUI with RS as moderate or greater; a slight impact of SUI on their overall quality of life. Female athletes managed SUI with containment products, fluid limitation, and timed voiding.
Gram and Bø 2020 [20]	Cross-sectional	n = 107	14.5 (1.6)	Rhythmic gymnastics	3	Urinary Incontinence short form (ICIQ-UI SF)	31.8	Triad-specific self-report questionnaire Beighton score	46.7% hypermobile; 9.3% disordered eating; 29.4% afraid of visible leakage; 14.7% afraid leakage would happen again; 69.1% had never heard about the pelvic floor.

* Mean (IQR); (IQR Interquartile range).

Table 2. Summary of participants' characteristics.

	Weight (kg)	BMI (kg/m^2)	Hours of Training/wk
Eliasson et al. [31]	50 (42–60) *	20.3 (19–23) *	-
Carls et al. [18]	-	-	-
Parmigiano et al. [19]		21.6 (2.8)	10.9 (4.0)
Fernandes et al. [32]	-	NP	-
Da Roza et al. [33]	55.0 (4.9)	20.4 (1.3)	11.3 (2.7)
Almeida et al. [34]	-	21.7 (2.6) **	19.0 (6.3)
Logan et al. [14]	-	-	-
Dobrowolski et al. [12]	-	21 (20–23) **	6 (4–6)
Gram & Bø [20]	-	18.9 (2.2)	15.7 (7.8)

* Mean (IQR); ** Median (IQR Interquartile range).

Our systematic review identified nine studies published between 2002 and 2020. The total sample was 633 female athletes, with an average age of 16.15 years, BMI ranging from 18.9 to 21.7 kg/m^2, and 6–19 h of training per week. We calculated a mean of prevalence of 48.58% for all the samples that were involved in different sports. Almost all study designs were cross-sectional (n = 8) where one had a pilot cross-sectional design. The risk of bias was assessed with the STROBE checklist for cross-sectional studies [29]. Figure 2 presents a heat map showing the grading of reporting completeness and quality for selected items according to the Strengthening the Reporting of Observational Studies in Cross-sectional studies. Eighty-seven percent of the articles explained the scientific background and rationale for the investigation and 62% stated specific objectives, including any specified hypotheses. Only 50% of the studies presented key elements of study design early in the paper and described the setting, locations, and relevant dates, including periods of recruitment, exposure, follow-up, and data collection. Study size was only explained in one study [31]. Clarity in defining all outcomes, exposures, predictors, potential confounders, and effect modifiers was applicable for 75% of the studies. Fifty percent of the included studies explained all of the statistical methods, including those used to control for confounding variables. Lastly, all studies summarized key results with reference to study objectives and discussed limitations of the study, taking into account sources of potential bias or imprecision.

3.3. Principle Findings

This systematic review identified a range of UI prevalence rates ranging from 18.2% to 80% and yielding a mean prevalence of 48.58%. In reports that assessed UI in one specific sport, the highest prevalence rates were found in trampolining (80%) followed by rope skipping (75%) and soccer (62.8%). On the other hand, the lowest rates of UI were found in practitioners of rhythmic gymnastics (31.8%).

The main outcome for assessing UI symptoms was the International Consultation on Incontinence short form questionnaire (ICIQ-SF), which was used in 5 of the 9 studies. Only one study used a quantitative measurement of UI through the pad-test [31]. Almost all studies included secondary assessments with questionnaires regarding the impact of UI on quality of life, specific type of urine loss, or associated pelvic floor dysfunctions such as fecal incontinence, sexual dysfunction, and pelvic organ prolapse. Only one study [31] measured muscular strength of the pelvic floor muscles. Of note, two of the included studies assessed female athlete triad risk factors including disordered eating behaviors [19,20]. Two studies assessed athletes' knowledge about pelvic floor muscle training (PFMT) [18,20]. A high percentage of adolescent female athletes (69% to 90%) had never heard of PFMT [18,20]. Moreover, 87% of adolescent female athletes stated they would not mention their UI symptoms to their coach [19].

Author/s		Recommendation	Not reported or unclear	Some information reported but insufficient	Clear and detailed information reported
		TITLE AND ABSTRACT			
	1.a	Indicate the study's design with a commonly used term in the title or the abstract			
	1.b	Provide in the abstract an informative and balanced summary of what was done and what was found			
		INTRODUCTION			
Background/rationale	2	Explain the scientific background and rationale for the investigation being reported			
Objectives	3	State specific objectives, including any prespecified hypotheses			
		METHODS			
Study design	4	Present key elements of study design early in the paper			
Setting	5	Describe the setting, locations, and relevant dates, including periods of recruitment, exposure, follow-up, and data collection			
Participants	6a	Give the eligibility criteria, and the sources and methods of selection of participants			
Variables	7	Clearly define all outcomes, exposures, predictors, potential confounders, and effect modifiers. Give diagnostic criteria, if applicable			
Data source/measurement	8	For each variable of interest, give sources of data and details of methods of assessment (measurement). Describe comparability of assessment methods if there is more than one group			
Bias	9	Describe any efforts to address potential sources of bias			
Study size	10	Explain how the study size was arrived at			
Quantitative variable	11	Explain how quantitative variables were handled in the analyses. If applicable, describe which groupings were chosen and why			
Stadistical methods	12.a	Describe all statistical methods, including those used to control for confounding			
	12.b	Describe any methods used to examine subgroups and interactions			
	12.c	Explain how missing data were addressed			
	12.d	If applicable, describe analytical methods taking account of sampling strategy			
	12.e	Describe any sensitivity analyses			
		RESULTS			
Participants	13.a	Report numbers of individuals at each stage of study—eg numbers potentially eligible, examined for eligibility, confirmed eligible, included in the study, completing follow-up, and analysed			
	13.b	Give reasons for non-participation at each stage			
	13.c	Consider use of a flow diagram			
Descriptive data	14.a	Give characteristics of study participants (eg demographic, clinical, social) and information on exposures and potential confounders			
	14.b	Indicate number of participants with missing data for each variable of interest			
Outcome data	15	Report numbers of outcome events or summary measures			
Main results	16.a	Give unadjusted estimates and, if applicable, confounder-adjusted estimates and their precision (eg, 95% confidence interval). Make clear which confounders were adjusted for and why they were included			
	16.b	Report category boundaries when continuous variables were categorized			
	16.c	If relevant, consider translating estimates of relative risk into absolute risk for a meaningful time period			
Other analyses	17	Report other analyses done—eg analyses of subgroups and interactions, and sensitivity analyses			
		DISCUSSION			
Key results	18	Summarise key results with reference to study objectives			
Limitations	19	Discuss limitations of the study, taking into account sources of potential bias or imprecision. Discuss both direction and magnitude of any potential bias			
Interpretation	20	Give a cautious overall interpretation of results considering objectives, limitations, multiplicity of analyses, results from similar studies, and other relevant evidence			
Generalisability	21	Discuss the generalisability (external validity) of the study results			
		OTHER INFORMATION			
Funding	22	Give the source of funding and the role of the funders for the present study and, if applicable, for the original study on which the present article is based			

≤2 articles
3-5 articles
7-8 articles

Figure 2. Assessment of reporting completeness and quality of included studies (STROBE).

4. Discussion

The aim of the present review was to systematically review the prevalence of UI among adolescent female athletes. Notably, we found a wide range of UI prevalence rates among young female athletes varying from 18% to 80%, with an average prevalence of UI symptoms in female adolescent athletes about 50%. Our results are slightly higher than the meta-analytic data presented by Teixeira et al. [16] for female athletes with an average age of 23.8 years, with a weighted average of 36% of UI prevalence. Additionally, our findings are significantly higher than the study by Hagovska et al. [34] who reported a UI prevalence of 14.3% in 503 adult female athletes (21.1 ± 3.6 years of age) who participated in high-impact sports. Notably, in the aforementioned study, the authors determined the impact of each sport activity based on metabolic intensity rather than on ground impact forces [17,35]. Along these lines, our data are in the range reported by Bø who reported a UI prevalence range between 10% and 55% in female athletes between 15 and 64 years of age [15]. Another review involving female athletes between 12 and 45 years [10], noted average prevalence rates varied from 1% to 42.2%

Our review included a total sample of 633 young nulliparous female athletes practicing a wide range of sports. Several studies included samples of athletes practicing different sports. We applied a classification of sport impact based on the study by Groothaussen and Siener [30] that has been specifically applied to the analysis of the impact of sports on the pelvic floor [7,10]. This impact classification is divided in 4 distinct groups: impact grade 3 (>4 times body weight, e.g., jumping); impact grade 2 (2–4 times body weight, e.g., sports involving sprinting activities and rotational movements), impact grade 1 (1–2 times body weight, e.g., such as lifting light weights); and impact grade 0 (<1 time body weight, e.g., swimming). The highest rates of UI in our sample were of grade 3 sports, which included jumping and landing actions (i.e., trampolining and rope skipping). Team sports graded 2 such as soccer, basketball, and track and field were found to display high prevalence rates as well. Impact activities such as running, jumping, and landing have been associated with increased intra-abdominal pressure in the pelvic organs and tissues [22,23]. The additional ground reaction forces placed on the continence structures may lead to displacement or insufficient counteractive muscle activity of the pelvic floor [22]. Another possible mechanism that may explain these prevalence rates is the relatively high metabolic intensity of selected sporting activities that contributes to the possible neuromuscular fatigue displayed by the pelvic floor muscles during training or competition [24]. Overall, the main characteristic of all sports performed in our sample was an impact grade between 2 and 3 [30].

The benefits of sports practice early in life are well established; however, young female athletes are not immune to suffering sport-related injuries or illness [36]. Particularly, the young female athlete can suffer from pelvic floor dysfunctions such as UI as well as pelvic pain and anal incontinence [6,34]. Almeida et al. [34] reported fecal incontinence, dyspareunia, and difficulty emptying the bladder in the female athletic group [34]. Low energy availability in female athletes has been noted as another health impairment that can impair pelvic floor function due to a constellation of hormonal, metabolic, and neuromuscular imbalances [26]. In this sense, Whitney et al. [37] found that female adolescent athletes (aged 15 to 19 years) with low energy availability had a higher prevalence of UI when compared with those with adequate levels of energy. Two studies included in our review assessed for the presence of eating disorders [19,20]. Parmigiano reported that 15% of their sample was at risk for suffering an eating disorder and Gram and Bø noted that 9.3% of adolescent rhythmic gymnasts were at risk for disordered eating [20]. In our review, the average volume of training and BMI of the sample ranged from 18.9 to 21.7 kg/m^2 and 6 to 19 h of training per week. Collectively, these observations suggest that the high volume and intensity of training along with low energy availability could be potential risk factors for developing UI in adolescent female athletes.

Bø and Sundgot-Borgen described that the presence of UI early in life is a strong predictor for UI later in life (ORR of 8.57) [7]. Moreover, leakage during sport practice has been shown to be a barrier to sports participation for young females [15,21]. Due to the observable health and fitness benefits of sports participation for girls and young women [36,38], additional studies are needed to improve our knowledge regarding pelvic floor dysfunction and implement effective preventative measures in active females. There is a lack of data targeting adolescent females investigating preventative, educational, and treatment modalities for UI. Given the high prevalence of UI in young female athletes and the lack of awareness of evidence-based preventative neuromuscular strategies such as PFMT and pelvic floor therapy [18,20,27], more studies are warranted. Pelvic physiotherapy has been found to be more effective in achieving continence in elite female athletes and pregnant athletes engaged in aerobic exercise compared to non-athletes [27]. For all these reasons, we suggest early screening with specific evaluation tools such as the pre-participation gynecological evaluation of female athletes proposed by Parmiagiano et al. [19] as well as the incorporation of specific neuromuscular training programs for the pelvic floor [13]. Increased awareness and educational programs targeting coaches and all female athletes regarding the pelvic floor musculature and specific dysfunctions such as UI are also warranted.

Limitations of this review are the small sample size, heterogeneity, and variability of outcome measures as well as the lack of reliable quantitative outcome measures for UI. The selected studies used validated questionnaires to assess urinary symptoms in young athletes. However, these questionnaires were validated in adult populations. More reliable diagnostic outcomes would improve the quality of the studies. In addition, the analysis of co-founding factors specific to the female adolescent athlete such as menstrual cycle and nutritional status would improve the quality of the studies. We recommend the use of the STROBE checklist for risk of bias study assessment to improve the scientific report of these studies and a classification of sport characteristics and impact, which would additionally improve their comparison and assessment. The development and validation of a specific questionnaire for assessing UI symptoms in adolescent females is warranted.

5. Conclusions

UI during exercise and sports is a concern for young female athletes. Our findings highlight a 48.8% prevalence rate among adolescent female athletes where practitioners of high-impact sports show the highest prevalence rates. Given the high prevalence of UI among adolescent female athletes involving impact sports graded 2 and 3, concerted efforts are needed to provide early education and implement prevention measures before young female athletes experience the burden of UI. Future research is needed to guide our understanding of the underlying physiopathology and unique characteristics of the adolescent female athlete's pelvic floor muscle activity during impact sports.

Author Contributions: Conceptualization, T.R.R. and I.C.-M.; methodology, C.G.-T.; software, C.G.-T.; validation, C.G.-T., I.C.-M. formal analysis, I.C.-M. and C.G.-T.; data curation, C.G.-T.; writing—original draft preparation, T.R.R.; writing—review and editing, T.R.R. and A.D.F.; supervision A.D.F. All authors have read and agreed to the published version of the manuscript.

Funding: This research received no external funding.

Institutional Review Board Statement: Not applicable.

Informed Consent Statement: Not applicable.

Data Availability Statement: Not applicable.

Conflicts of Interest: The authors declare no conflict of interest.

References

1. Haylen, B.T.; De Ridder, D.; Freeman, R.M.; Swift, S.E.; Berghmans, B.; Lee, J.; Monga, A.; Petri, E.; Rizk, D.E.; Sand, P.K.; et al. An International Urogynecological Association (IUGA)/International Continence Society (ICS) joint report on the terminology for female pelvic floor dysfunction. *Int. Urogynecol. J.* **2010**, *21*, 5–26. [CrossRef] [PubMed]
2. Aoki, Y.; Brown, H.W.; Brubaker, L.; Cornu, J.N.; Daly, J.O.; Cartwright, R. Urinary incontinence in women. *Nat. Rev. Dis. Prim.* **2017**, *3*. [CrossRef] [PubMed]
3. Minassian, V.A.; Drutz, H.P.; Al-Badr, A. Urinary incontinence as a worldwide problem. *Int. J. Gynecol. Obstet.* **2003**, *82*, 327–338. [CrossRef]
4. Almousa, S.; Bandin Van Loon, A. The prevalence of urinary incontinence in nulliparous female sportswomen: A systematic review. *J. Sports Sci.* **2019**, *37*, 1663–1672. [CrossRef] [PubMed]
5. De Araujo, M.P.; Sartori, M.G.F.; Girão, M.J.B.C. Incontinência de atletas: Proposta de novo termo para uma nova mulher. *Rev. Bras. Ginecol. e Obstet.* **2017**, *39*, 441–442.
6. Bø, K.; Borgen, J.S. Prevalence of stress and urge urinary incontinence in elite athletes and controls. *Med. Sci. Sports Exerc.* **2001**, *33*, 1797–1802. [CrossRef]
7. Bø, K.; Sundgot-Borgen, J. Are former female elite athletes more likely to experience urinary incontinence later in life than non-athletes? *Scand. J. Med. Sci. Sports* **2010**, *20*, 100–104. [CrossRef]
8. Pires, T.; Pires, P.; Moreira, H.; Viana, R. Prevalence of Urinary Incontinence in High-Impact Sport Athletes: A Systematic Review and Meta-Analysis. *J. Hum. Kinet.* **2020**, *73*, 279–288. [CrossRef]
9. Almousa, S.; Bandin van Loon, A. The prevalence of urinary incontinence in nulliparous adolescent and middle-aged women and the associated risk factors: A systematic review. *Maturitas* **2018**, *107*, 78–83. [CrossRef]
10. de Mattos Lourenco, T.R.; Matsuoka, P.K.; Baracat, E.C.; Haddad, J.M. Urinary incontinence in female athletes: A systematic review. *Int. Urogynecol. J.* **2018**, *29*, 1757–1763. [CrossRef]
11. Rubilotta, E.; Balzarro, M.; D'Amico, A.; Cerruto, M.A.; Bassi, S.; Bovo, C.; Iacovelli, V.; Bianchi, D.; Artibani, W.; Agrò, E.F. Pure stress urinary incontinence: Analysis of prevalence, estimation of costs, and financial impact. *BMC Urol.* **2019**, *19*, 44. [CrossRef] [PubMed]
12. Dobrowolski, S.L.; Pudwell, J.; Harvey, M.A. Urinary incontinence among competitive rope-skipping athletes: A cross-sectional study. *Int. Urogynecol. J.* **2020**, *31*, 881–886. [CrossRef] [PubMed]
13. Rial, T.; Chulvi-Medrano, I.; Faigenbaum, A.D.; Stracciolini, A. Pelvic Floor Dysfunction in Women. *Strength Cond. J.* **2020**, *42*, 82–91. [CrossRef]
14. Logan, B.L.; Foster-Johnson, L.; Zotos, E. Urinary incontinence among adolescent female athletes. *J. Pediatr. Urol.* **2018**, *14*, 241.e1–241.e9. [CrossRef]
15. Bø, K. Urinary incontinence, pelvic floor dysfunction, exercise and sport. *Sports Med.* **2004**, *34*, 451–464. [CrossRef]
16. Teixeira, R.V.; Colla, C.; Sbruzzi, G.; Mallmann, A.; Paiva, L.L. Prevalence of urinary incontinence in female athletes: A systematic review with meta-analysis. *Int. Urogynecol. J.* **2018**, *29*, 1717–1725. [CrossRef]
17. Hagovska, M.; Svihra, J.; Bukova, A.; Horbacz, A.; Svihrova, V. The impact of physical activity measured by the International Physical Activity questionnaire on the prevalence of stress urinary incontinence in young women. *Eur. J. Obstet. Gynecol. Reprod. Biol.* **2018**, *228*, 308–312. [CrossRef]
18. Carls, C. The prevalence of stress urinary incontinence in high school and college-age female athletes in the midwest: Implications for education and prevention. *Urol. Nurs.* **2007**, *27*, 21–24.
19. Parmigiano, T.R.; Zucchi, E.V.M.; de Araujo, M.P.; Guindalini, C.S.C.; de Aquino Castro, R.; Di Bella, Z.I.K.D.J.; Girão, M.J.B.C.; Cohen, M.; Sartori, M.G.F. Pre-participation gynecological evaluation of female athletes: A new proposal. *Einstein* **2014**, *12*, 459–466. [CrossRef]
20. Gram, M.C.D.; Bø, K. High level rhythmic gymnasts and urinary incontinence: Prevalence, risk factors, and influence on performance. *Scand. J. Med. Sci. Sports* **2020**, *30*, 159–165. [CrossRef]
21. Casey, E.K.; Temme, K. Pelvic floor muscle function and urinary incontinence in the female athlete. *Phys. Sportsmed.* **2017**, *45*, 399–407. [CrossRef] [PubMed]
22. Moser, H.; Leitner, M.; Eichelberger, P.; Kuhn, A.; Baeyens, J.P.; Radlinger, L. Pelvic floor muscle displacement during jumps in continent and incontinent women: An exploratory study. *Neurourol. Urodyn.* **2019**, *38*, 2374–2382. [CrossRef] [PubMed]
23. Leitner, M.; Moser, H.; Eichelberger, P.; Kuhn, A.; Baeyens, J.P.; Radlinger, L. Evaluation of pelvic floor kinematics in continent and incontinent women during running: An exploratory study. *Neurourol. Urodyn.* **2018**, *37*, 609–618. [CrossRef] [PubMed]
24. Ree, M.L.; Nygaard, I.; Bø, K. Muscular fatigue in the pelvic floor muscles after strenuous physical activity. *Acta Obstet. Gynecol. Scand.* **2007**, *86*, 870–876. [CrossRef]
25. Kruger, J.A.; Dietz, H.P.; Murphy, B.A. Pelvic floor function in elite nulliparous athletes. *Ultrasound Obstet. Gynecol.* **2007**, *30*, 81–85. [CrossRef]
26. Rial, T.; Stracciolini, A. Pelvic floor dysfunction in female athletes: Is relative energy deficiency in sport a risk factor? *Curr. Sports Med. Rep.* **2019**, *18*, 255–257.
27. Sorrigueta-Hernández, A.; Padilla-Fernandez, B.-Y.; Marquez-Sanchez, M.-T.; Flores-Fraile, M.-C.; Flores-Fraile, J.; Moreno-Pascual, C.; Lorenzo-Gomez, A.; Garcia-Cenador, M.-B.; Lorenzo-Gomez, M.-F. Benefits of Physiotherapy on Urinary Incontinence in High-Performance Female Athletes. Meta-Analysis. *J. Clin. Med.* **2020**, *9*, 3240. [CrossRef]

28. Moher, D.; Liberati, A.; Tetzlaff, J.; Altman, D.G. Preferred Reporting Items for Systematic Reviews and Meta-Analyses: The PRISMA Statement. *PLoS Med.* **2009**, *6*, e1000097. [CrossRef]
29. von Elm, E.; Altman, D.G.; Egger, M.; Pocock, S.J.; Gøtzsche, P.C.; Vandenbroucke, J.P. The Strengthening the Reporting of Observational Studies in Epidemiology (STROBE) statement: Guidelines for reporting observational studies. *Lancet* **2007**, *370*, 1453–1457. [CrossRef]
30. Groothausen, J.; Siemer, H.; Kemper, H.C.G.; Twisk, J.; Welten, D.C. Influence of peak strain on Lumbar Bone Mineral Density: An analysis of 15-year physical activity in young males and females. *Pediatr. Exerc. Sci.* **1997**, *9*, 159–173. [CrossRef]
31. Eliasson, K.; Larsson, T.; Mattsson, E. Prevalence of stress incontinence in nulliparous elite trampolinists. *Scand. J. Med. Sci. Sports* **2002**, *12*, 106–110. [CrossRef] [PubMed]
32. Fernandes, A.; Fitz, F.; Silva, A.; Filoni, E.; Filho, J.M. Evaluation of the Prevalence of Urinary Incontinence Symptoms in Adolescent Female Soccer Players and their Impact on Quality of Life. *Occup. Environ. Med.* **2014**, *71*, A59–A60. [CrossRef]
33. Da Roza, T.; Brandão, S.; Mascarenhas, T.; Jorge, R.N.; Duarte, J.A. Urinary Incontinence and Levels of Regular Physical Exercise in Young Women. *Int. J. Sports Med.* **2015**, *36*, 776–780. [CrossRef] [PubMed]
34. Almeida, M.B.A.; Barra, A.A.; Saltiel, F.; Silva-Filho, A.L.; Fonseca, A.M.R.M.; Figueiredo, E.M. Urinary incontinence and other pelvic floor dysfunctions in female athletes in Brazil: A cross-sectional study. *Scand. J. Med. Sci. Sports* **2016**, *26*, 1109–1116. [CrossRef]
35. Hagovska, M.; Švihra, J.; Buková, A.; Hrobacz, A.; Dračková, D.; Švihrová, V.; Kraus, L. Prevalence of urinary incontinence in females performing high-impact exercises. *Int. J. Sports Med.* **2017**, *38*, 210–216. [CrossRef]
36. Carder, S.L.; Giusti, N.E.; Vopat, L.M.; Tarakemeh, A.; Baker, J.; Vopat, B.G.; Mulcahey, M.K. The Concept of Sport Sampling Versus Sport Specialization: Preventing Youth Athlete Injury: A Systematic Review and Meta-analysis. *Am. J. Sports Med.* **2020**, *48*, 2850–2857. [CrossRef]
37. Whitney, K.E.; Holtzman, B.; Parziale, A.; Ackerman, K.E. Urinary incontinence is more common in adolescent female athletes with low energy availability. *Orthop. J. Sports Med.* **2019**, *7*, 2325967119S0011. [CrossRef]
38. Eime, R.M.; Young, J.A.; Harvey, J.T.; Charity, M.J.; Payne, W.R. A systematic review of the psychological and social benefits of participation in sport for children and adolescents: Informing development of a conceptual model of health through sport. *Int. J. Behav. Nutr. Phys. Act.* **2013**, *10*, 98. [CrossRef]

MDPI
St. Alban-Anlage 66
4052 Basel
Switzerland
Tel. +41 61 683 77 34
Fax +41 61 302 89 18
www.mdpi.com

Journal of Functional Morphology and Kinesiology Editorial Office
E-mail: jfmk@mdpi.com
www.mdpi.com/journal/jfmk

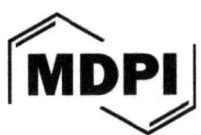

www.ingramcontent.com/pod-product-compliance
Lightning Source LLC
LaVergne TN
LVHW070619100526
838202LV00012B/685